Praises for The Bragg Healthy Lifestyle

Thanks to the ageless Bragg Health Books, they were our introduction to healthy living. We are very grateful to you and your father. – Marilyn Diamond, Co-Author "Fit For Life" Best Seller – 40 weeks

Bragg Healthy Lifestyle, Breathing, vinegar drink and brisk walking (3x daily) for 20 minutes after meals, helped eliminate my diabetes! My whole body, circulation, feet and eyes all improved. Thank you, may God continue to bless Bragg Crusade. – John Risk, California

The Bragg Healthy Lifestyle, the vinegar drink and fasting has changed my life! I lost weight and my energy levels went through the roof. I look forward to my fasting days. I think better and am a better husband and father. Thank you Patricia and Paul, this has been a great blessing in my life. Also, we enjoyed your health sharing at our "AOL" Conference. – Byron H. Elton, VP Entertainment, Time Warner AOL

For over 40 years I've followed Bragg Healthy Lifestyle – it teaches you how to take control of your health and build a healthy future. – Mark Victor Hansen, Co-Producer, "Chicken Soup for Soul" Series

I love the books and your ACV! It has made such a difference in my life and to my family. For over a year I was having such terrible skin issues – my skin was peeling like I had a sunburn all the time, I had rosacea and adult acne. Two dermatologists were of no help. No medications, face wash or creams were helping. After meeting you and using your ACV as a tonic for my face, it has cleared up to where you would never know I had a problem. I use the ACV as a drink 4 times a day. I lost 6 pounds in 2 weeks following your simple instructions on the Bragg Healthy Lifestyle found in Bragg ACV Book. Thank you for coming into my life when I needed help! Love and Blessings! – Becky, Boca Raton, Florida

Thank you Patricia for our first meeting in London in 1968. You gave me your Fasting Book, it got me exercising, brisk walking and eating more wisely. You were a blessing God-sent. – Rev. Billy Graham

Bragg Books were my conversion to the healthy way. – James Balch, M.D., Co-Author "Prescription for Nutritional Healing"

Improper breathing is a common cause of ill health. Changing your breathing patterns can affect and improve you mentally, emotionally and physically. – Andrew Weil, M.D.

b

Praises for This Super Power Breathing Book and The Bragg Healthy Lifestyle

I'm a big Paul Bragg fan and I daily use Bragg Liquid Aminos on my food. I even take it with me when I travel for my seminars, I wouldn't be without it! The world and I are blessed with Bragg Health Teachings!
– Anthony "Tony" Robbins • *www.AnthonyRobbins.com*

In Medical School I read Dr. Bragg's Health Books. They changed my way of thinking and the path of my life. I founded Omega Institute.
– Stephan Rechtschaffen, M.D. • *www.Eomega.org*

Paul Bragg inspired me many years ago with the "Miracle of Fasting" and with his philosophy on health. His daughter Patricia is a testament to the ageless value of living the Bragg Healthy Lifestyle. – Jay Robb, Author of "The Fruit Flush"

I have known Bragg Health Books for over 40 years. They are a blessing to me and my family and to all who read them to help make this a healthier world. – Pastor Mike MacIntosh, Horizon Christian Fellowship, San Diego, CA • *HorizonSD.org*

Thanks to Bragg "Miracle of Fasting" and "Healthy Lifestyle" books, we're healthy, fit and singing better and staying younger than ever!
– The Beach Boys • *www.BeachBoysFanClub.com*

Your dad, Dr. Paul Bragg IS the FATHER of the natural health industry and the entire natural health movement. Everything that has been done in natural health and physical culture since has been based on the pioneering vision and principles articulated by Dr. Bragg. He gave us all our health direction!
– Dr. William Wong • *www.DrWong.us*

I am following The Bragg Healthy Lifestyle which I heard of through a friend. Your books are motivators and have blessed my health and my life and are making the best perfect gifts for my family and friends. – Delphine, Singapore

I had the opportunity to sit next to Patricia on a flight from Dallas to L.A. Her honesty about my weight and health really inspired me to make a life change. One year later, I am 85 lbs. lighter and heart rate cut almost in half. Patricia you helped save my life! – Mike Ableman, Texas

How I beat cancer, obesity, diabetes, strep and three herniated disks and excruciating pain? The answer was changing to the Bragg's Healthy Lifestyle and doing the Super Power Breathing Exercises. It changed and saved my life! I had full recovery and also lost 70 lbs. I received a new life and that is just the beginning because my manhood returned that was lost to diabetes – now that's exciting! On my trip to Honolulu, I visited the famous free Bragg Exercise Class at Waikiki Beach. I became so regenerated with a wonderful new viewpoint towards living the Bragg Healthy Lifestyle that I now live in Hawaii. I'm invigorated with new energy for life and living! My new purpose for living is to help others reclaim their health rights! I want the world to join The Bragg Health Crusade. I am deeply thankful to Paul and Patricia for my new healthy life!
– Len Schneider, Hawaii

Warm wishes all the way from Malaysia to express my sincere gratitude to both of you for sharing your precious health secrets of health and youthfulness with The Bragg Healthy Lifestyle Living!
– Marilyn Lim, Sarawak, Malaysia

I've experienced a beautiful, remarkable, spiritual and physical awakening since reading Bragg Books. I'll never be the same again.
– Sandy Tuttle, Painesville, Ohio

Daily we get letters at our Santa Barbara headquarters. We would love to hear from you on any blessings, healings and impact on your life you experienced after following The Bragg Healthy Lifestyle. It's all within your grasp to be in top health! By following this book, you can reap Super Health and a happy, long, vital life! It's never too late to begin – see page 192-193, the study they did with people in their 80's and 90's and the amazing results that were obtained! You can receive miracles with nutrition, exercise and some fasting! Start now!

Daily our prayers & love go out to you, your heart, mind & soul.

Patricia and *Paul C. Bragg*

Miracles can happen every day through guidance and prayer! – Patricia Bragg

BRAGG PHOTO GALLERY

PATRICIA & PAUL C. BRAGG, ND, PhD.'s
Dynamic Daughter & Father are World Health Crusaders

HEALTH IS HERE

During the past century, Bragg Live Food Products developed and pioneered the very first line of Health Foods, from vitamins and minerals to raw nuts, seeds, and sun-dried fruits. This included more than 365 health products – *"one for each day of the year!"* says daughter Dr. Patricia Bragg.

"Thanks for The Bragg Healthy Lifestyle that you shared with me and you are sharing with millions of others worldwide."
– John Gray, Ph.D., Author

Picture from
People Magazine August, 1975

Patricia and father, Paul on world trip in 1950's, during stop in Tahiti.

"You have recharged me with joy, hope, love and encouragement, which poured from your words. I am now fasting and using ACV. You have certainly improved my life!"
– Marie Furia, New Jersey

Patricia Bragg stands on her father's stomach. Paul's stomach muscles are so strong he can lift Patricia up and down!

E

PAUL BRAGG, ND, PhD.
HEALTH CRUSADER
Life Extension Specialist and
Originator of Health Food Stores

I love Bragg Products! My family uses Bragg Liquid Aminos spray on popcorn for a treat. You will see it recommended in many of the recipes in my books.
– Marilu Henner, Actress & Health Book Author
• *marilu.com*

Actress Donna Reed saying "Health First" with Paul Bragg.

Dr. Paul C. Bragg (right) Creator Health Food Stores, Pioneer Life Extension Specialist, with his prize student Jack LaLanne. Paul started him on the royal road to health over 81 years ago!

Paul C. Bragg spent much of his time at the Hollywood Studios meeting with top Stars and motion picture industry executives, giving health lectures and private consultations. Dr. Bragg was Hollywood's first highly respected, health, fitness and nutrition advisor to the Stars.

Paul C. Bragg with Gary Cooper, famous American film actor, best known for his many Western films.

Paul Bragg with famous Hollywood Actress Gloria Swanson, who was leading starlet in 20s, 30s and 40s. Gloria became a Bragg Health Devotee at 18 and she often would Health Crusade with Bragg during the 1950s.

Maureen O'Hara & Paul Bragg. This Irish film actress & singer was best noted for playing in "Miracle on 34th Street" and "The Quiet Man".

PAUL C. BRAGG, ND, PhD.
STAYING HEALTHY & FIT

I'd like to thank you for teaching me how to take control of my health! I lost 55 pounds and I feel "great"! Bragg books have showed me vitality, happiness and being close to Mother Nature. You both are real "Crusaders for Health for the World". Thanks!
– Leonard Amato

Paul Bragg owes his powerful body and superb health to living exclusively on live, vital, healthy, organic rich foods.

Paul C. Bragg and daughter Patricia were my early guiding inspiration to my health career and health education.
– Jeffery Bland, Ph.D., Famous Food Scientist

Paul Bragg in Tahiti (1920's) gathering tropical papaya fruit.

Bernarr Macfadden & Paul Bragg

A thousand happy Bragg Health Students enjoy hiking, exercise and fresh air on the trail to Mount Hollywood (above Griffith Observatory) in beautiful California, summer of 1932.

Paul C. Bragg at Regent's Park, London

PHOTO GALLERY PAUL & PATRICIA BRAGG

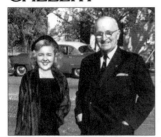

Patricia with 33rd President Harry S. Truman at his home in Independence, Missouri.

Paul Bragg, Creator of Health Food Stores, with his prize student Jack LaLanne, who thanks Bragg for saving his life at 15.

Dr. Patrica Bragg with Dr. Jeffrey Smith. He is leader in getting GMO's out of US foods. See GMO video by Jeffrey Smith and narrated by Lisa Oz (Dr. Oz's wife) on web: *GeneticRouletteMovie.com*

Patricia visiting with Steve Jobs at his home in Palo Alto during the Thanksgiving Holidays.

"I've been reading Bragg Books since high school. I'm thankful for the Bragg Healthy Lifestyle and admire their health crusading for a healthier, happier world."
– Steve Jobs, Creator & CEO – Apple Computer

Paul in 1920 with his swimming & surfing friend, Duke Kahanamoku, Waikiki Beach, Diamond Head.

Patricia, Paul Bragg and Mrs. Nadine Kahanamoku. (Nadine is Patricia's Godmother)

Dr. Earl Bakken with Patricia. He's famous for inventing the first transistor pacemaker. His firm Medtronic, developed it and a resuscitator for fixing ailing hearts that have and are saving thousands of lives. Dr. Bakken lives in Hawaii & is a big Bragg Liquid Aminos fan.

"I cannot remember a time when the Golden Rule* was not my motto and precept, the torch that guided my footsteps." – J.C. Penney

H *** The Golden Rule:** Do unto others as you would have them do unto you.

J.C. Penney & Patricia ➡ exercising. They walked often in Palm Springs when he and his wife visited in the winter to enjoy the warm desert sunshine.

HEALTH CRUSADING TO HOLLYWOOD STARS

Patricia with friend Actress Jane Russell. Famous Hollywood Star of 40s to 60s.

Jane Wyatt learning about health with Paul C. Bragg.

Mickey Rooney with Paul. Rooney is an American film actor and entertainer. He has won multiple awards and has had one of the longest careers of any actor to age 93.

Paul C. Bragg exercising with Actress Helen Parrish.

"Thank you Paul & Patricia Bragg for my simple, easy-to-follow Healthy Lifestyle. You make my days healthy!" – Clint Eastwood, Academy Award Winning Film Producer, Director, Actor and Bragg follower for over 60 years

Paul Bragg and Donna Douglas, one of Hollywood's most beautiful, talented and best Health Girls. She played the part of "Elly-May" in the *Beverly Hillbillies*, which became one of the longest-running series in television history and was the #1 show in America in its first 2 years.

> **Life is a Precious Miracle Minute by Minute Year by Year!**

Paul with James Cagney, American film actor. He won major awards for wide variety of roles. The American Film Institute ranked Cagney 8th among the Greatest Male Hollywood Stars of All Time.

Patricia with Conrad Hilton

◄ Hotel founder, Conrad Hilton with Patricia Bragg, his Healthy Lifestyle Teacher. *"I wouldn't be alive today if it wasn't for the Braggs and their Bragg Healthy Lifestyle!"*. – Conrad Hilton

"Thank you for your website. What a wealth of info to learn about how to live and eat healthy. Many Blessings." – Michel & Mary, CA

I

PHOTO GALLERY

PAUL C. BRAGG, ND, PhD.
PROMOTES HEALTH & FITNESS!

Paul C. Bragg leading an exercise class in Griffith Park, Hollywood, CA – circa 1920s.

Bragg Healthy Lifestyle works Miracles! – Jack LaLanne

Paul and Patricia love swimming & being active.

Friend and Paul Bragg doing handstand at the beach.

Paul running on Coney Island, New York, where he was a member of the Coney Island Polar Bear Club, known for Cold Water Swimming, 1930s.

TV Hulk Actor Lou Ferrigno gives thanks to Bragg Books. Lou went from puny to become Super Hulk. ➡

"I lost 102 lbs. with Bragg Apple Cider Vinegar and Bragg Healthy Lifestyle and have kept it off for over 15 years, staying away from white flour, sugar and other processed foods." – Dee McCaffrey, Chemist & Diet Counselor, Tempe, Arizona

Lou & Patricia in Chicago Health Freedom Expo.

DR. PATRICIA CONTINUING THE HEALTH CRUSADE!

Dear Friends – you cannot know how greatly you have impacted my life and some of my friends! We love your Bragg Health Books, teachings and products and are now living healthier, happier lives. Thanks!
– Winnie Brown, Arizona

Jack LaLanne with Patricia Bragg

Mother Nature Loves US!

Patricia Bragg with Bill Galt inspired by Bragg Books and founded Good Earth Restaurants.

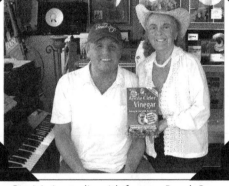

Patricia in studio with famous Beach Boy Bruce Johnson, Bragg follower over 35 years. He played for her his latest records.

Patricia with Jean-Michel Cousteau, Ocean Explorer & Environmentalist. *OceanFutures.org*

Enjoy a Lifetime of Radiant Health

Patricia with Jack Canfield, Bragg follower, Motivational Speaker and Co-Producer of *Chicken Soup for the Soul* Series.

Patricia with Astronaut Buzz Aldrin, celebrating over 46 years since pilot of Apollo 11 first landed on the moon.

Famous Hollywood Actress Cloris Leachman (89 years young), ardent health follower who sparkles with health and vitality says, *"Bragg Miracle of Fasting Book is a miracle . . . it cured my asthma, my years of arthritis and many other health problems. I praise Paul and Patricia daily for their Health Crusading!"*

PAUL & PATRICIA BRAGG
HEALTH CRUSADING

Patricia with Jay Robb

Paul C. Bragg on the Merv Griffin Show, 1976

Paul Bragg inspired me many years ago with the Miracle of Fasting Book and his pioneering philosophy on health! His daughter Patricia is a testament to the ageless value of living The Bragg Healthy Lifestyle. – Jay Robb, Author of *The Fruit Flush*

During the 50-plus years Patricia worked with her father, she was right beside him, assisting him on Bragg Health Crusades worldwide. They were a great team, when you looked at them, you would see only two people headed in the same healthy direction!

I am a big fan of Paul Bragg. I fast and use the Bragg Aminos daily on my food. I even take it with me when I travel for my seminars, I wouldn't be without it! The world and I are blessed with the health teachings of Paul and Patricia Bragg! – Anthony "Tony" Robbins

❀ **Roses are God's Autograph of Beauty, Fragrance and Love** ❀

Paul – London Bragg Health Crusade

Paul & Daughter Patricia, Royal Hawaiian, Honolulu.

Actor Arthur Godfrey with Patricia, in Honolulu celebrating his 79th Birthday.

Health Crusaders Paul C. Bragg and daughter Patricia traveled the world spreading health, inspiring millions to renew and revitalize their health.
Bragg Mottos:
3 John 2 and Genesis 6:3

100 YEAR HISTORY OF BRAGG HEALTH BOOKS & PRODUCTS

Four Generation Health Food COOK BOOK — $3.00

PHILOSOPHY OF SUPER-HEALTH

BRAGG APPLE CIDER VINEGAR SYSTEM — Learn these powerful health qualities...

Natural Apple Cider Vinegar is proving to be one of the greatest aids to health and long life known to science. It is an entirely natural substance, produced by powerful enzymes (life chemicals). Cider Vinegar is used in many ways, both internally and externally.

BRAGG TOXICLESS DIET — BODY PURIFICATION & HEALING SYSTEM

Paul and Patricia are passionate, dedicated in spreading message of health to world.

Dr. Patricia Bragg carries on her father's Health Legacy that he started over 100 years ago.

View on Web: 100th Anniversary Party www.bragg.com

BRAGG LIQUID AMINOS
Delicious Seasoning with 16 Essential Amino Acids, still available worldwide.

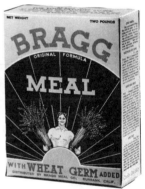

BRAGG MEAL CEREAL
Bragg was first to put 7 grains together for a delicious hot cereal.

BRAGG SANSAL
A great Salt Substitute. This product was approved by Los Angeles Heart Assoc.

BRAGG SPRINKLE
Delicious Herb Seasoning. Started 1931 – the first with 24 Organic Herbs & Spices.

BRAGG ORGANIC MINT TEA
First Organic Herb Teas in America

"Our lives have completely turned around! Our family is feeling so healthy, we must tell you about it."– Gene & Joan Zollner, parents of 11, Washington

PHOTO GALLERY

CELEBRATING YEARS OF HEALTH CRUSADING

HALL of LEGENDS
Dr. Patricia Bragg

PALM SPRINGS WALK OF STARS

Paul C. Bragg with daughter, celebrating over 50 years of Bragg Health Products, Books & Crusading worldwide, spreading Health around the world.

1962

Here is Dr. Patricia with BRAGG STAR
See more pictures on Bragg.com/blog

Natural Foods Expo in Anaheim with 65,000 attendees from around the world honored Dr. Patricia Bragg and her father Paul C. Bragg as treasured Health Food Industry Legends.

BRAGG's 100th Anniversary Celebration

Mrs. Jack LaLanne

Katy Perry's Parents

Dr. Patricia Bragg

2012

Patricia, Staff & 1,000 Friends celebrated our 100 years of Bragg Healthy Products, Books & Health Crusading! We are proud Pioneers in this Big Health Industry that is helping to keep the world healthier! With Blessings of Health, Peace & Love to You!

Patricia

See Slide-Video Show of Party at: bragg.com/party.htm

Bragg Hawaii Exercise Class was founded by Worldwide Health Crusader and Fitness Legend, Dr. Paul C. Bragg. He wanted to create a dynamic, Free Community Exercise Class, and he often taught these classes himself for many years. Dr. Patricia Bragg continues her father's health legacy by supporting the Bragg Exercise Class and participates in the class whenever she is in Hawaii.

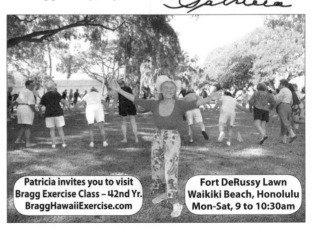

Patricia invites you to visit
Bragg Exercise Class – 42nd Yr.
BraggHawaiiExercise.com

Fort DeRussy Lawn
Waikiki Beach, Honolulu
Mon-Sat, 9 to 10:30am

"Please make a record of your family history & background. Take pictures – make your own 'Photo Gallery'. Take videos – make movies of your children, your spouse, your mother and father, family gatherings, etc. These memories are precious and important to save for future generations." – Patricia Bragg

BRAGG
SUPER POWER
BREATHING

For Our Life, Super Health,
High Energy & Longevity

PAUL C. BRAGG, N.D., Ph.D.
LIFE EXTENSION SPECIALIST

and

PATRICIA BRAGG, N.D., Ph.D.
HEALTH CRUSADER & LIFESTYLE EDUCATOR

Blessings
of
Health

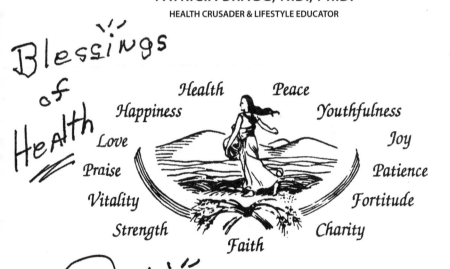

Health   *Peace*
Happiness   *Youthfulness*
Love   *Joy*
Praise   *Patience*
Vitality   *Fortitude*
Strength   *Charity*
Faith

Patricia

It's FREE – JOIN & ENJOY
Bragg Health Crusades for a 100% Healthy World for All!

HEALTH SCIENCE
Box 7, Santa Barbara, California 93102 USA

World Wide Web: www.bragg.com

Notice: Our writings are to help guide you to live a healthy lifestyle and prevent health problems. If you suspect you have a medical problem, please seek alternative health professionals to help you make the healthiest informed choices. Diabetics should fast only under a health professional's supervision! If hypoglycemic, add spirulina or barley green powder to liquids when fasting.

BRAGG
SUPER POWER
BREATHING

PAUL C. BRAGG, N.D., Ph.D.
LIFE EXTENSION SPECIALIST

and

PATRICIA BRAGG, N.D., Ph.D.
HEALTH CRUSADER & LIFESTYLE EDUCATOR

Health Science, Box 7, Santa Barbara, California 93102
Telephone (805) 968-1020, FAX (805) 968-1001
e-mail address: books@bragg.com

Quantity Purchases: Companies, Professional Groups, Churches, Clubs, Fundraisers, etc. Please contact our Special Sales Department.

To see Bragg Books and Products on-line, visit our Website at: www.bragg.com

 This book is printed on recycled, acid-free paper, which saves thousands of trees.

- REVISED AND EXPANDED -

Twenty-fifth Printing MMXVI
ISBN: 978- 0-87790-120-4

Library of Congress Cataloging-in-Publication Data on file with publisher

Published in the United States
HEALTH SCIENCE, Box 7, Santa Barbara, California 93102 USA

PAUL C. BRAGG, N.D., Ph.D.
World's Leading Healthy Lifestyle Authority

Paul C. Bragg's daughter Patricia and their wonderful, healthy members of the Bragg *Longer Life, Health and Happiness Club* exercise daily on the beautiful Fort DeRussy lawn, at famous Waikiki Beach in Honolulu, Hawaii. View club exercising *BraggHawaiiExercise.com*. Membership is free and open to everyone to attend – Monday through Saturday, 9 to 10:30 am – for Bragg Super Power Breathing and Health and Fitness Exercises. On Saturday there are often health lectures on how to live a long, healthy life! The group averages 50 to 75 per day, depending on the season. From December to March it can go up to 125. Its dedicated leaders have been carrying on the class for over 42 years. Thousands have visited the club from around the world and have carried the Bragg Health and Fitness Crusade to friends and relatives back home. When you visit Honolulu, Hawaii, Patricia invites you and your friends to join her and the club for wholesome, healthy fellowship. She also recommends visiting the outer Islands (Kauai, Hawaii, Maui, Molokai) for a fulfilling, healthy vacation.

To maintain good health, normal weight and increase the good life of radiant health, joy and happiness, the body must be exercised properly (stretching, walking, jogging, running, biking, swimming, deep breathing, good posture, etc.) and nourished wisely with healthy foods. – Paul Bragg, ND, PhD.

iii

WE NEED YOUR SUPPORT!

Help us make a huge impact and join us as a Health Crusader!
Support The Bragg Health Crusades to Continue to Spread Paul C. Bragg's Teachings Around the World

For over 80 years we have been sharing Paul C. Bragg's teachings on healthy living worldwide! Millions are following the Bragg Healthy Lifestyle principles and their lives have been changed forever! Everyday people send us letters, e-mails and call, saying – *"Paul Bragg saved my life!"*

Former U.S. Surgeon General, Dr. C. Everett Koop said, "Paul Bragg did more for the Health of America than any one person I know of."

OUR MISSION: To inspire and educate people of all ages throughout the world to adopt a Healthy Lifestyle through optimal Nutrition, Exercise, Positive Attitudes and Spiritual Wellness.

Paul C. Bragg, N.D., Ph.D.
Originator of Health Stores
Life Extension Specialist
Health Crusader to the World

If your life has been touched and helped by Bragg Health Teachings, please help us carry on The Bragg Legacy in this 21st Century and beyond. Bragg is very committed to this effort and as part of its core values wants to give back to communities in this meaningful way. Bragg contributes generously to many non-profits and schools every year, and your additional support would make an even bigger impact in our communities. Your tax deductible donation to *Bragg Health Foundation* will support our mission to continue the Bragg Message of Health worldwide and inspire future generations.

The non-profit and philanthropic work of *The Bragg Health Foundation* funds *The Bragg Health Crusades,* community health, health education to schools, adults, and free training and health publications to military service and their families to help handle stress. Bragg helps conduct health outreach to youth in schools through our new *BraggHealthKids.org* program, also organic gardening teaching programs and helps sponsor Health Science Research and provides scholarships to worthy students pursuing natural health science professions.

Please join us in sharing The Bragg Health Legacy!

(Please see next page for more information)

Bragg Outreach to Schools

iv   Patricia Bragg lecturing at
Bragg Health Seminars

Organic Gardening
Teaching Programs

Bragg Scholarships

SHARE OUR DREAM WITH NEW HEALTH VISION

Health Crusades Entrance

The Bragg Health Foundation is located on a beautiful 120 acre Campus and Organic Farm on the Coast of Santa Barbara, California. Patricia Bragg and the Directors of Bragg Health Foundation have designated this as the future site of the greatest living tribute to the life of Paul C. Bragg. The Bragg Health Foundation is becoming a world center for organic, healthy lifestyle education and research. (See our *Mission, Purpose & Vision for the Future* video on *BraggHealth.org*)

You can also be part of Paul Bragg's lasting legacy by having your name inscribed upon one of the educational nature walks or inspirational walls of the Bragg Health Foundation Campus and Organic Farm. Or you may want to have your name inscribed in the Grand Entrance or a room in the Bragg Memorial Library or Health Education Center or you can sponsor the Health Teaching DVDs to schools.

Your name can be part of your own legacy, as you will be recognized for generations to come as a great Health Crusader because of your financial support of these wonderful health projects. When thousands of visitors see your name each year, they will know that you helped make a difference in the world. **Visitor's Circle & Fountain**

Some Special Health Projects You Can Partner with us:

❑ *Bragg Health Kids* Programs, DVDs ❑ Organic Teaching Gardens
❑ Scholarships for Naturopathic Students ❑ Healthy Ageing & Longevity
❑ Paul C. Bragg Library & Rose Gardens ❑ Bragg Nature & Farm Walks
❑ Special Health Events & Programs ❑ Military Health Programs

— — — — — — — — — *MAKE COPY AND MAIL* — — — — — — — — —

YES! I would like to help support Bragg Health Crusades by making a contribution to the Bragg Health Foundation, a 501(c)(3) non-profit foundation, tax ID# 30-0033989 Your contributions are tax deductible.

❑ Enclosed is my tax-deductible gift of $_____ ○ Check ○ VISA ○ MC ○ Discover
   ○ $25 ○ $50 ○ $100 ○ $250* ○ $500* ○ $1,000* ○ $2,500* ○ $_____
❑ Please send me info on where my name can be permanently inscribed at Bragg Center.

My gift is in honor/memory of _____

Please send notice of this gift to (name & address):_____

_____

Credit Card Number:_____

Signature:_____

Card Expires: _____ / _____
month / year

Your Name   PLEASE PRINT

Address   Apt. No.

City   **State**   **Zip**

Phone ( )   **e-mail**

If giving by check, please make check payable to: **Bragg Health Foundation**
Mail To: Box 7, Santa Barbara, CA 93102 USA • (805) 968-1020

For more info check out our web: www.BraggHealth.org
Spreading health worldwide since 1912
Donate today and receive a Bragg gift bag of Bragg books and products!

*For contributions of $250 or above you are eligible for an exclusive "Naming Opportunity" on one of these areas – Nature Walk, Apple Orchard or Adopt-A-Tree. (Donor Plaques available)

V

BRAGG HEALTH FOUNDATION
Promoting Health and Wellness Worldwide

BRAGG COMMUNITY HEALTH

Bragg Health Foundation conducts free Health Lectures and produces and distributes a variety of educational publications featuring Health, Wellness and Longevity. Lectures are held throughout the community, at local Libraries, Schools, Churches and Community Centers, along with Cooking, Exercise and Fitness demonstrations, and all are offered at no cost to the schools, etc. and all attendees.

THE BRAGG ORGANIC ORCHARD

The Bragg Award Winning Organic Farm distributes free organic apples and fruits to schools and food service organizations to provide nutritional healthy options. A portion of the harvest is used in production of our world famous Bragg Organic Apple Cider Vinegar.

THE BRAGG HEALTH KIDS PROGRAM

The Bragg Health Foundation is proud to provide wisdom on Nutrition, Wellness and Health Education designed and loved by both kids and parents. Bragg Health Kids Program centers its fun teaching curriculum on this wise Bragg Health Motto:

'You Are What You Eat, Drink, Breathe, Think, Say and Do!'

We are providing an educational online program that provides lessons on the importance of living a 100% Healthy Lifestyle. With engaging videos, interactive exercises and varied health education information and activities to inspire all children to enjoy living a healthy lifestyle.

BRAGG Health Foundation

Dr. Patricia Bragg,
ND, PhD, ScD.
Chairman of the Board,
Bragg Health Foundation

President and CEO,
Bragg Live Food Product

Dr. John Westerdahl,
PhD, MPH, RD, CNS
Director of the
Bragg Health Foundation

Director of Health Science,
Bragg Live Food Products

A 501(c)3 nonprofit organization, Bragg Health Foundation operates to benefit the greater good of community under the guidance of our Board of Directors, Chairman of the Board, Executive Director and dedicated staff, all knowledgeable and skilled in nonprofit leadership, operations and health programs.

To make a secure on-line donation today please visit: Donate.BraggHealth.org

vi

Super Power BREATHING

To preserve health is a moral and religious duty, for health is the basis for all social virtues. We can't be as useful when not well.
– Dr. Samuel Johnson, Father of Dictionaries

Contents

Breathing is the greatest pleasure in life – it gives life! – Papini, 1881-1956

Shallow breathing helps to increase symptoms of almost every known sickness!

A fool thinks he needs no advice, but a wise man listens & learns from others.
– Proverbs 12:15

Contents

One of the most tragic things about human nature is that all of us tend to put off living. We are dreaming of some magical rose garden over the horizon – instead of enjoying the roses that are blooming outside our windows today. – Dale Carnegie

Learning is finding out what you already knew. Doing is demonstrating that you know it! Teaching is reminding others that they know it just as well as you! You are all learners, doers and teachers! – Richard Bach

We need to protect our planet, our wildlife, soil, land, air and water!

Contents

When you live The Bragg Healthy Lifestyle you can help activate your own powerful internal defense arsenal and maintain it at top efficiency. But, bad or sloppy breathing habits make it harder for your body to fight off illness.

Contents

Contents

*Kindness should be a frame of mind in which we are alert to every chance:
to do, to give, to share and to be kind and loving.* – Patricia Bragg, ND, PhD.

We shall never know all the good that a simple smile can do. – Mother Teresa

xi

Contents

The best service a book can render you is, to impart truth,
but to make you think it out for yourself. – Elbert Hubbard

God gave you a gift of 86,400 seconds today (24 hours).
Have you used one to say "thank you? – William Arthur Ward

May you always have an angel by your side,
watching out for you in all the things you do.

No matter what your sense of direction, you'll never lose your way.
Your angel will always keep you on the right path. – Suzanne Siegel Zenkel

Contents

I conceive that a knowledge of books is the basis on which all other knowledge rests. – George Washington, First U.S. President, 1789-1797

Contents

Contents

We all grow healthier in nature, gentle sunshine and love! – Patricia Bragg, ND, PhD.

Today, give a stranger one of your smiles.
It might be the only sunshine he sees all day. – H. Jackson Brown, Jr.

Contents

 Bragg Healthy Lifestyle Plan

- *Read, plan, plot, and follow through for supreme health and longevity.*
- *Underline, highlight or dog-ear pages as you read important passages.*
- *Organizing your lifestyle helps you identify what's important in your life.*
- *Be faithful to your health goals everyday for a healthy, long, happy life.*
- *Where space allows we have included "words of wisdom" from great minds to motivate and inspire you! Please share your favorite sayings with us.*
- *Write us about your successes following The Bragg Healthy Lifestyle.*

Visit *bragg.com* and send free Bragg Health Musical E–Cards from our web to friends!
Also follow Patricia and get Bragg Health Messages on *twitter.com/PatriciaBragg*
Watch Bragg Videos on *YouTube.com/PatriciaBragg*

DO YOU SHOW SIGNS OF PREMATURE AGEING?

Is everything you do a big effort?

•

**Have you started to lose your skin tone?
Your muscle tone? Your energy? Your hair?**

•

**Do small things irritate you?
Are you forgetful?   Confused?**

•

Is your elimination sluggish?

•

Do you have allergies? Joint pains?

•

Do your feet hurt?

•

Do you have aches and pains?

•

**Do you get out of breath
when you run or climb stairs?**

•

How limber is your back and body?

•

How well do you adjust to cold and heat?

•

**Ask yourself these important questions:
Am I healthy and happy?
Do I seem to be slipping and
not quite like myself anymore?
If the answer to these questions are "Yes,"**

START TODAY
Living The Bragg Healthy Lifestyle!

Loss of Teeth

HAIR OF • THINNING

FADING OF • SIGHT

SALIVARY GLANDS SHRINK

LOSS OF HEARING

HIGH BLOOD PRESSURE

STIFFENING OF JOINTS

xvii

He who understands and follows Mother Nature walks with God.

❧ *Decades of Amazement as Life Rolls By* ❧

Where did our years go? They went by so fast.
When we're young they seem to cra-a-wl,
With each decade, they fly past!

At 29 we're the center; At 30 we feel supreme
But 40 strikes terror; Life's not what it seems.
By 50 we've reached maturity; At 60 we accept seniority.
When we're filled with excitement of creative living,
There's no room for depression and despair!

But at 65, wisdom that comes from experience
Then takes over and we learn to accept ourselves as we are.
Each new day is a gift to be treasured,
Enabling us to go far!

At 75, life is for the living
But it is through our sharing, loving and giving
that we reach the Stars of Joy, Peace
and the Possibilities of Eternity!

– by Ruth Lubin, 88 years young & going strong,
who started writing poetry & sculpturing at 80!
PS: Ruth is a fan of the Bragg Healthy Lifestyle for over 58 years!

❤ WITH LOVE PROMISE YOURSELF ❤

- *Promise yourself to be so strong that nothing can disturb your peace of mind.*

- *To talk health, happiness and prosperity to every friend person you meet.*

- *To make your friends feel that they are special & appreciated.*

- *To look at the sunny side of life & everything & make your optimism come true.*

- *To think only of the best, to work only for the best and expect only the best.*

- *To be just as enthusiastic about the success of others as you are about your own.*

- *To forget the mistakes of the past and press on to the greater achievements of the future.*

- *To be too large for worry, too noble for anger, too strong for fear & too happy to permit the presence of trouble & fear.*

- *To give so much time to the improving yourself that you have no time to never criticize others.*

- *To wear a cheerful expression at all times and give a smile to every living creature you meet.*

– Christian D. Larson
Author & Influential Leader

Chapter 1

Super Power Breathing For Super Energy

Do You Know How to Breathe?

The breath of life means exactly what it says: To breathe is to live; not to breathe is to die. A human can exist without food for weeks, go without water for days, but one can't exist for more than a few minutes without air!

This fact is so obvious and breathing is so automatic that most people take it for granted. *Yet, do you really know how to breathe?* Stop and think about it. Do you really know how your lungs function? Do you use these marvelous organs to their fullest? The way you use your lungs controls your life, your health, your looks, your energy, your resistance to disease – your very life span!

Super Power Breathing – The Path To High Vibration Energy Living

As health specialists with over a century of combined effort, we have developed techniques for measuring mental and physical energy in humans. Everyone lives at a certain rate of vibration. The human body is capable of reaching a high vibration energy level; unfortunately many never master what it takes to achieve this. Why? Because only a few know how to generate, utilize and replenish their full capacity of body and mind energy!

High vibration energy people are doers and achievers. They display seemingly inexhaustible vitality and stamina, creative power and/or athletic ability of the highest quality. They never seem to tire. They perform mental and physical tasks without strain or excessive emotion. To high vibration achievers, everything seems easy and effortless because they have more vital power!

Breathing is the most basic of bodily functions!

The Bragg Super Power Breathing habit of taking longer, slower, deeper breaths helps to produce more energy and a more vital, youthful, longer life for you!
– Paul C. Bragg, ND, PhD, Life Extension Specialist, Originator of Health Stores

High Vibration Energy Produces Achievers

This natural energy produces contented people who see the humorous side of life: full of personal magnetism and enthusiasm. High vibration energy people are a joy to be with because they have happy dispositions. They are free from depressions and mental blocks, and are well-adjusted people who enjoy more fulfilling, healthy and happy lives. What is their secret? How do they live at a superior rate of high vibration energy? The answer is simple: such people consume large amounts of oxygen. They breathe deeply and fully, utilizing every square inch of their lung capacity. Ample oxygen combined with a healthy lifestyle does bring miracles.

The more oxygen you breathe into your lungs, the more energy you will have. This creates a higher rate of vibration. It is very much like a fire in an open burning fireplace, the more oxygen the fire gets, the brighter it will burn! The less oxygen it gets, the less heat and more unwanted smoke it generates – and soon the fire dies.

Most Live at Low to Medium Vibration

People who live at a low to medium rate of vibration attain limited levels of vitality, both mentally and physically. While they may have a capacity for work and play, they aren't capable of the sustained effort achieved by those who have high vibration energy. Low to medium vibration energy people easily tire and lack endurance, particularly when under stress. Exhaustion induced by tension and strain forces this type of person to stop, rest and sadly even give up.

People living even at a medium vibration rate simply don't get enough vital oxygen to give them that extra push to keep going under physical, mental or emotional pressures. Under extreme pressure they *run out of gas* and lack the high vibration energy that deep power breathing and healthy living provides to make this additional effort.

Our life-sustaining lungs fuel us with oxygen. We breathe in and out 22,000 times per day – processing about 300 cubic feet of air – just the amount needed to oxygenate 2,400 gallons of blood that is pumped through the heart daily.

Super Power Breathing Increases Energy

At age 16, my father, Paul C. Bragg, was diagnosed with a *hopeless* case of tuberculosis. Yet by age 18 he was cured and became a successful athlete. During those two years he was under the care of the great Swiss physician Dr. August Rollier. This wise doctor gave Dad a new lease on life with a regimen of all-natural healing methods. Using only pure distilled water, good nutrition, an apple cider vinegar drink, sunshine, fresh air, deep breathing and regular exercise, his body was able to cure itself with healthy natural living. After being healed, my father made a life-long pact with God to share his healthy lifestyle message with millions worldwide and he has!

Paul C. Bragg became a great-great-grandfather. He could out last most people half his age or less in any competition requiring energy and stamina. He easily typed for hours without mental or physical fatigue. He enjoyed hiking, jogging, biking, swimming, lifting weights, surfing, playing tennis and the challenge of climbing the highest mountains around the world.

Benefits of Effective Super Power Breathing

It is through breathing that we take in oxygen to fuel our minds and bodies. The more fuel we have, the better we function. The more effectively we breathe, the more effectively we live. Benefits of effective breathing include:

- increased oxygen intake
- balance of the emotions
- relief of stress
- relaxation of the body
- calming of the mind
- enhanced mental focus, clarity & creativity
- increased oxygenation of the blood, tissues, muscles & organs

Super Power Breathing *can make your life-force stronger, calmer and smarter, which is wonderful when you stop and think about it – something so simple that can be so powerfully helpful and healthful to your total well-being!*

We can live for weeks without food, days without water, but only minutes without breathing. This tells us that breath and breathing is the element that's truly supplying our life-force on a minute by minute basis. I hope your starting to see why breathing is so absolutely important to the body. – NaturalNews.com

Count your blessings one by one and you will see what the Lord has done! I give thanks daily for all the Miracle Blessings I receive daily. – Patricia Bragg, ND, PhD.

Listen for your angel's voice in music, in kind words, in walks, loving thoughts, flowers, nature, and precious memories.

It's Never Too Late for You to Improve!

My father kept himself at a high rate of mental and physical vibration by supplying his body with the correct fuel: natural, healthy "live" foods and, above all, ample super power oxygen! He continually helped people in all walks of life – musicians, singers, writers, artists, doctors, lawyers, athletes, office workers and homemakers – to achieve a superior state of high vibration energy so they could enjoy Bragg Healthy Living. The basic source of super-oxygen-vibration is knowing how to deeply fill your lungs with oxygen. Everyone is born with this capacity, but unfortunately only a few retain this deep breathing habit naturally throughout life like athletes and singers do!

Whatever your age, it's never too late to learn how to increase your energy with the Bragg System of Super Power Breathing. After faithfully following the breathing exercises in this book, you too can soon learn how to fill your lungs with energy-producing, super power oxygen. You will enjoy the thrill of this great oxygen stimulation. It's far more potent than any toxic artificial stimulants such as alcohol, coffee, tea, cola and soft drinks and drugs. Plus oxygen has no side effects! In fact, deep oxygen stimulation can add up to a longer, healthier and fuller, happier lifetime.

The Miracle Surge of the Second Wind Helps Olympic Champions Win!

Why can't some get their *second wind*? It is because they are not using the full capacity of their miracle lungs for energy-producing oxygen. That is the big difference between the person who lives at the high vibration level and those who draw on only a medium rate of vibration. At a high rate of vibration, when you consume your full quota of oxygen, you are able to get your *second wind*. You feel stronger than when you started your effort. This miracle *second wind* is what makes high achievers, champion athletes, statesmen and women, writers, singers, actors, dancers and go-getters are equally high achievers.

Healthy Mind Habit: *Wake up and say, "Today I am going to be happier, healthier and wiser in my daily living! I am the captain of my life and am going to steer it to living a 100% healthy lifestyle!" Fact is happy people look younger & have fewer health problems!* – Patricia Bragg, ND, PhD., Pioneer Health Crusader

4

When you learn to use the full capacity of your lungs through the Bragg System of Super Power Breathing, you will experience this wonderful stimulation of the *second wind*. Just when you think you have run out of energy, this sudden renewal of strength occurs! This is an experience truly difficult to describe. When you feel you cannot take another step, that your brain power is all gone, that your thinking is befuddled, then suddenly a great surge of energy courses through your entire body. You soon feel as fresh as, or even stronger than when you started! What a tremendous sensation! When you do this breathing correctly you experience this amazing *second wind!* **Many Olympic champions won their gold medals using Bob Anderson's wise help – the world's leading stretching coach (Stretching book on *amazon.com*) teaches Bragg Super Power Breathing at seminars worldwide.**

Shallow Breathing Causes Premature Ageing

Regrettably, even the people who live at a medium rate of vibration are in the minority. In our modern world, most people are only half alive, existing merely at a very low rate of physical and mental vibration! Look around you – this includes people of all ages – from the early teens to the late 80's (if they live that long). Babies use their lungs as Mother Nature and God intended, but soon they acquire the unnatural, lazy, *civilized* habit of shallow breathing and begin to use only the top part of their lungs.

Shallow breathing starves the body of the oxygen it needs to be vitally alive! That's why there are so many people – from teenagers to oldsters – crowding doctors' offices, clinics, sanitariums, hospitals and convalescent homes. They drag themselves through life, seeking imaginary quick-fixes from artificial remedies in the form of laxatives, painkillers, tonics, sleeping pills and other popular, advertised over-the-counter drugs.

Breathing is our connection to life, through the body and heart, leading us to a wholeness of being and giving us spirit for living life to its fullest. – S. Hainer, M.S.

I cannot overstate the importance of the habit of quiet prayer and meditation for more health of body, mind, and spirit.
"In quietness shall be your strength." – Isaiah 30:15

The natural healing force within you is the greatest force in getting well.
– Hippocrates, Father of Medicine, 400 B.C.

Oxygen-starved people are usually nervous and suffer from unnecessary worries as well as physical ills! Millions go to bed exhausted and wake up tired. They suffer from headaches, constipation, indigestion, muscular aches and pains, stiff joints, sore backs and feet, painful teeth and receding gums, poor eyesight and hearing, loss of memory, inflamed throats and respiratory ailments such as bronchitis, asthma, sinus infections and emphysema.

These health miseries and the loss of healthy bodily functions (which are often attributed to *ageing)* plague millions, sadly can take them to an early grave! They suffer and die needlessly – simply because they don't live a healthy lifestyle and most importantly, learn to breathe deep and fully! It seems incredible, but with Super Power Breathing miracles happen! Prove it to yourself! **Life and health are priceless and should be treasured!**

Faith and Vision Create Miracles

Those happy, healthy, strong, vigorous people – who accomplish greatness – are those of faith that possess a deep spiritual philosophy. They believe that their lives are protected by a Power greater than their own. They believe there is a destiny that guides their lives. Nothing can stop them! Following the wise Laws of God and Mother Nature you can accomplish great miracles!

(Xerox page, cut out Patricia's Angel Strip, for you to fold and keep in wallet.)

Angel to Protect & Guide You

Here's your own "Pocket Angel" to be with you 24/7 night and day to guide, protect, and show you right from wrong, and help you heal your life – physically, mentally, emotionally and spiritually with Angel Love.

They that wait upon the Lord
shall renew their strength;
They shall mount up
with wings as eagles;
They shall run, and not be weary;
And they shall walk, and not be faint.

Chapter 2

Oxygen and Your Health
Oxygen Starvation

Suppose you are very hungry and sit down to enjoy a well-planned, nourishing meal . . . but as soon as you have eaten only a few bites of the food, someone snatches it away and tells you that you can't have any more! What would you think of the food-snatcher?

This is exactly what you do to yourself when you shallow breathe as most people do, using only 1/4 to 1/3 of your lung capacity! This starves your body more than if you were depriving it of food! You are slowly robbing your body of its most vital, invisible nourishment – oxygen!

Oxygen is essential to the ionization process, in which food molecules are broken down into nutrients suitable for the body's vital needs. Without sufficient oxygen your body cannot properly utilize the food you eat and drink, no matter how basically nourishing the food may be.

With an insufficient supply of life-giving oxygen, your blood slowly becomes saturated with poisonous carbon dioxide and other toxic wastes. It transports these toxins throughout your body (collecting more enroute), thereby suffocating your cells (also dulling brain cells), instead of rejuvenating them with sufficient life-giving oxygen!

Your brain, which requires three times more oxygen than the rest of your body, suffers first. This warning was stated by top child specialist with delinquent children:

> *"55% of the delinquent behavior in minors can be attributed to oxygen starvation."* Philip Rice, M.D.

Oxygen starvation is caused by shallow breathing, sedentary habits and the lack of exercise and fresh air! Educators who are alarmed about the decrease in the average student's IQ would do well to promote school physical education, exercise, sports and open windows! Tests and analyses are not brain food, but life-giving oxygen is!

Rhythmic Breathing brings more air and oxygen into lungs and bloodstream.

Life-Giving Oxygen – Invisible Staff of Life

You can perform a simple demonstration by lighting two candles and placing them side by side, a few inches apart. Now partially cover one candle with a glass . . . watch how small and pale this flame becomes. If you cover the candle completely with the glass, the flame will go out in a few seconds. That is what happens in your body when you deprive it of life-giving oxygen.

THE HEART AND BLOOD VESSEL CIRCULATORY SYSTEM

Head

Right arm and hand

Left arm and hand

Aorta

Right lung

Left lung

Right auricle
Portal circulation
Vena cava

Left auricle
Right ventricle
Left ventricle
Heart

Right kidney

Left kidney

Legs and feet

Whole Body View of Blood Circulatory System

The diagram shows vital, life-giving blood being pumped from right side of the heart through the lungs where **oxygen** is absorbed into the blood, then on to the left side of the heart, then through the system back to the right side of the heart again. All the blood from the digestive system goes through the portal veins; thus through the liver and continues its miracle circulation throughout the entire body.

When we inhale, oxygen from the air we breathe is diffused through membranes and into red blood cells. The oxygen-rich blood then circulates throughout the body and finds tissues in need of oxygen. – NaturalNews.com

Your heart and body takes care of you and keeps you alive – be good to it!

Oxygen Powers Your Miracle Human Machine

The human body is a miracle intricate mechanism for the production of mental and physical energy. Oxygen, the invisible staff of life is this mechanism's power source. Your body begins to function with your first breath and continues until your last! How well it functions depends on your lifestyle and how well you supply it with oxygen!

As in any heat or combustion engine, **oxygen is essential to the production of energy in your body.** Every flame consists of the union of oxygen with other elements. The gasoline that fuels your car, the natural gas or coal in a heater or furnace and the wood in a fireplace or stove all contain latent energy. This energy cannot be released to produce the heat or power until its elements are broken down and united with life-giving oxygen!

This human body process is called metabolism. The food you eat contains latent energy, but it's of absolutely no use to you without oxygen. To determine the general health of our bodies, we can test the rate of our basal metabolism. This rate is determined in a laboratory by measuring the oxygen we use while our body is resting.

As long as you live, the body mechanism operates for you continuously. Even while asleep, your lungs, heart, kidneys, liver and other major organs, as well as circulatory and nervous systems, must continue 24/7 to function! Amount of energy you need depends upon your mental and physical activities! **The release of energy you need depends upon your intake of oxygen and your general health. Champion athletes are deep breathers!**

Oxygen is Carried by the Bloodstream

Every one of the over 90 trillion cells in your body demands a continuous flow of life-giving oxygen in order to stay alive, do its job and remain healthy! This oxygen supply is carried in your bloodstream by the red blood cells. There are millions of these red cells in every drop of your blood.

I love Bragg Books. "The Miracle of Fasting" is so popular and loved in Russia and Ukraine. I give thanks for my health and energy. I just won famous Honolulu Marathon with all-time women's record! – Lyubov Morgunova, Moscow, Russia

---

Bragg Super Power Breathing helps make the weak strong & athletes champions. – Bob Anderson, famous stretching coach to Olympic champions • stretching.com

Blood – Your Miracle River of Life!

The blood circulates in an average network of around 60,000 miles of blood vessels that reach every cell in the body, from those of the heart itself to the top of the scalp and to the tips of the fingers and toes. The average individual has about five to six quarts of blood circulating throughout their vast miracle body network at all times.

During rest or inactivity the blood makes on average one round trip per minute. During strenuous activity or exercise, however, it may make as many as eight or nine round trips per minute in order to supply the necessary fuel and oxygen for increased energy, and to help remove waste products and toxins from the body.

The blood vessels that carry blood from the heart are known as arteries. Those that return blood to the heart are veins. Both vary greatly in size and are organized just like streams, brooks and creeks flowing into a river, which joins a larger river. **Your body is a working miracle machine.**

The smallest blood vessels are called capillaries. They are so tiny that most are visible only under a microscope! Through these capillaries the last of the food and oxygen is given off and the return trip is made via the veins, which carry the oxygen-depleted blood and toxic wastes back to the heart for purification. Enroute to the heart, however, most of the water-soluble wastes are transferred to the kidneys for elimination through the urine. Poisonous carbon dioxide gas, a major residue of energizing oxidation, is brought back to the heart to be expelled through the lungs in breathing.

Super Power Breathing Detoxifies and Purifies Your Blood

The carbon dioxide collected from all parts of the body gives blood a blueish color when it is returned through the veins to the heart. There it enters the right auricle, the heart's upper chamber. After the auricle fills with blood, the valve into the right ventricle (lower chamber) opens, allowing the blood to pass into the ventricle. When the valve closes, the ventricle's strong muscles contract, sending blood to the lungs.

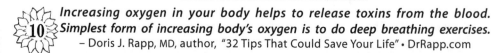

Increasing oxygen in your body helps to release toxins from the blood. Simplest form of increasing body's oxygen is to do deep breathing exercises.
– Doris J. Rapp, MD, author, "32 Tips That Could Save Your Life" • DrRapp.com

As blood travels through the capillary network in the lungs' air sacs, it discharges its load of carbon dioxide. It turns a healthy, bright red again as it absorbs the vital, life-giving oxygen before it immediately returns to the hearts left auricle. From there the blood flows into the left ventricle and by valve action is pumped vigorously into the body's largest artery, the aorta. Leaving the aorta, the blood then travels throughout the body via a vast arterial network – taking its life-giving oxygen and nutrients to every body cell to keep you healthy!

It is the shorter or *lesser* circulation – from the heart to the lungs and back – that is so vital to detoxifying and purifying the bloodstream! If the lungs are only partially filled with air, then only part of the bloodstream can be cleansed. The blood which passes through the capillaries of empty air sacs cannot get rid of its carbon dioxide waste and cannot pick up oxygen! So, instead of carrying a full quota of life-giving oxygen back to the cells of the body, the bloodstream returns with a mixture of fresh oxygen and a residue of toxic poisons. As this sluggish process continues, the proportion of carbon dioxide buildup increases, causing health problems!

How Oxygen Supports Body Detoxification

Health in the human body depends to a large degree on how efficiently nutrients can be absorbed and utilized at the cellular level, as well as how effectively the toxins and wastes can be removed! Cellular waste is removed from the body in several ways. Part of the waste is dissolved in water and transported to the kidneys and liver for filtration. It is then eliminated through the urine and bowels. Toxins are also excreted from the body through perspiration.

However, some of the most toxic poisons in the body can only be "burnt up" and neutralized through oxidation. This is the job of oxygen-rich red blood cells that circulate from the lungs and into the deeper organs and glands of the body. See web: *NaturalNews.com.*

Blood is the miracle river of life that flows through the human body. We cannot live without blood! The heart pumps blood to all our body's cells, supplying them with needed nutrition and oxygen.

Shallow Breathers Self-Poison Themselves

When you are a shallow breather, you don't change the air at the base of your lungs, where two-thirds of your lung capacity is located. When you return impure blood to your body, the ill effects are compounded because your blood cannot perform properly. It is difficult for blood that's loaded with poisonous wastes to transport relatively small amount of oxygen which it absorbs; it's even harder for it to carry necessary nourishment from food. An inadequate oxygen supply impairs your body's ability to break down food into digestible elements. This slows all bodily function! This is why deep breathing is so vitally important for health!

With wrong diet and shallow breathing, the organs of elimination are overworked and underfed! But accumulating wastes must go somewhere. Some are discharged into sweat glands. This toxic overload produces unpleasant body odors! Other toxic wastes end up deposited as heavy mucus into sinus cavities, lungs and bronchial tubes. Some line the passages of ears, eyes, nose and throat, as well as along the digestive tract. Deposits of hardened wastes in moveable joints can cause pressure on nerves, creating painful warning signals. **Pain is Mother Nature's flashing red warning signal that something is wrong in your body!** This pain warning should be respected with corrective measures taken right away – not repressed by painkilling drugs full of both known and unknown side-effects!

Shallow breathers actually poison themselves by robbing their bodies of sufficient oxygen! This is auto-intoxication (self-poisoning). They are slowly suffocating and dying in their own body wastes and poisons. **Pneumonia is a shocking example; body and lungs fill up and drown in their own toxins and mucus.**

Consider this: if someone tried to force you to kill yourself by taking shallow breaths, what would you do? You'd fight back! In defiance, you would breathe deeply, cleansing your blood and entire miracle body system to give your body more life, energy and super health!

Shallow breathers, unfortunately, only bring in 10% of fresh air with each breath. Deep breathers however bring in 80% fresh air to energize their body!
– Readers Digest Book of Facts (www.rd.com)

Oxygen Deprived Cells Show Cancer Connection

Healthy cells in the body are aerobic, meaning they require adequate levels of oxygen for cellular respiration and growth! When cells are deprived of oxygen for any reason, decay sets in and the cells can mutate or die.

Dr. Otto Warburg, 1931 Nobel prize winner, discovered a close connection between oxygen and cancer. His studies showed that **the primary cause of cancer is directly related to oxygen-deprived cells!** In fact, he found that cancer cells are anaerobic and actually thrive in an oxygen-deficient environment.

Warburg also discovered that a slightly alkaline pH in the body meant higher levels of oxygen uptake. Now, having low blood oxygen level is normal clinical finding sadly for people with chronic diseases! (*NaturalNews.com*)

Increasing Your Body's Oxygen Naturally

Aerobic Exercise increases level of oxygen in the body. Exercising as brisk walking (page 187), swimming, cycling, dancing and the mini-trampolining (rebounder) helps heart and lungs to work more efficiently! When lungs give heart the oxygen it needs it doesn't have to overwork and not as susceptible to heart attacks! Exercise for 30 minutes a day – 5 times a week is recommended.

Deep Breathing in a slow and relaxed way oxygenates and relaxes the body! Deep coordinated inhalation brings oxygen to tissues, while deep exhalation helps move wastes from the body! Without proper breathing coordination, built-up tensions, etc. cause breathing to become erratic and shallow. By consciously replacing that habit by deeper breathing, you can bring benefits to both mind and body!

Fill Your Lungs with Super, Life-Giving Oxygen

Breath Expansion Test: *Before beginning Bragg Super Power Breathing Program, perform this simple test. Exhale fully and measure deflated chest with a tape measure. Take a deep breath and measure again. After a month of practicing these exercises, take test again. You will be amazed by how much more super life-giving oxygen fills your lungs as you practice Bragg Super Power Breathing.*

Oxygen is one of the primary catalysts for energy and optimal health in the human body! – NaturalNews.com

A raw food diet is highest in oxygen. Eat organic fresh fruits, green vegetables and sprouted seeds and nuts. Live fruits, green vegetables and sprouted/soaked seeds and nuts are composed of water, which is hydrogen and oxygen and mostly oxygen by weight. The green in vegetables is chlorophyll which is very close in atomic structure to human blood. Chlorophyll has a magnesium atom and human blood differs only with an iron atom. With enzymes from raw food the magnesium ion is changed to an iron one making blood that can transport oxygen for human use instead of CO_2 for plant use.

An oxygen-depleting diet consists of cooked foods, red meat, sugar, saturated fats, white bread, processed and frozen foods, and carbonated beverages! Switching to an oxygen-rich diet often brings fast energy and a more vibrant body, skin and positive attitude! Choose foods rich in chlorophyll as dark green leafy foods like spinach, collards, chard, kale, mustard greens, spirulina, chlorella and blue-green algae. Also try juicing them with veggies.

Adequate Hydration. Drinking enough water daily is essential not only for utilization of oxygen in the body, but also for transporting the blood and other bodily fluids. Without adequate water, all bodily functions are diminished, including cellular respiration and removal of toxins and metabolic wastes. Drinking 8 glasses distilled water is necessary to get the full benefits of oxygenation.

Massage increases circulation which carries more oxygen to individual cells of the body. Massage enhances all essential body processes by opening the passageways of liquid and energy movement within the body.

Ozone air-purifying machines are extremely effective in destroying and eliminating airborne pollutants, fumes, cigarette smoke, chemicals, odors, fungi, mold, bacteria, and viruses from the air. For more information see web:
Breathing.com/articles/oxygen-increase.htm

---

*The life-force and oxygen within me is feeding my strength –
the strength of my body, soul and mind.* – Paul C. Bragg, ND, PhD.

Shallower, more rapid nervous breathing results in insufficient vital oxygen reaching the brain. – Susan Smith Jones, PhD, Author "Health Bliss" – amazon.com

---

Your heart rate varies with your breathing: it slows down when you exhale and speeds up when you inhale. – Neil F. Gordon, "Breathing Disorders" – amazon.com

---

There is no wealth greater than the health of the body. – The Bible

Chapter 3

The Way You Breathe Affects Your Life

When You Breathe Deeply and More Fully You Live Healthier, Happier, Longer Lives

When you pump a generous flow of oxygen into your body, every cell becomes more alive! This enables the four main *motors* of your body – the heart, lungs, liver and kidneys – to operate and perform better. Your miracle-working bloodstream purifies and cleanses every part of the body, including itself. This eliminates toxic wastes as Mother Nature planned and then fuel (food) and vital oxygen are carried to every cell in your miracle body.

With ample oxygen your muscles, tendons and joints function more smoothly. Your skin becomes firmer and more resilient and your complexion clearer and glowing. You will radiate with greater health, energy and super well-being for a long life!

With Super Power Breathing your brain becomes more alert and your nervous system functions better. You become free from tension and strain because you can easily take the stresses and pressures of daily living. Your emotions come under your control. You feel joyous and exuberant. If negative emotions such as anger, hate, jealousy, greed or fear intrude, expel them with positive thinking and slow, concentrated, relaxed deep breathing!

The deep breather enjoys more peace of mind, tranquility and serenity! In India, the great teachers practice deep, full breathing as the first essential step towards higher spiritual development. You attain higher concentration in meditation by taking long, slow, deep breaths. Deep breathing stimulates your brain cells and promotes new brain cell growth, as Salk Scientist explains on next page.

I command my life force to breathe deeply for vibrant, super health. Oxygen is the vital, precious, invisible staff of life. – Paul C. Bragg, ND, PhD.

Life is in the breath. He who half breathes, half lives! – Old Proverb

Super Deep Breathing Improves Your Brain

The person who breathes deeply and fully thinks more clearly and sharply! Oxygen stimulates your logic and intelligence. The more deeply and fully you breathe, the greater your power of concentration and the more your creative mind will assert itself. You will also develop greater extrasensory perception within your body, especially the brain. Scientists at the *Salk.edu* for Biological Studies, La Jolla, CA, now know that adults do generate new brain cells in the hippocampus, an area in the brain which is responsible for learning and memory. Deep breathing nourishes and fine-tunes the brain and entire body!

Bragg Super Power Breathing will help to constantly rejuvenate you to a higher energy vibration of living! The more fully and deeply you breathe, the further you will travel to higher levels on the physical, mental and spiritual planes. **Now sit back, relax, close your eyes and for 3 to 5 minutes enjoy some slow, deep breathing!**

Correct Breathing Can Reduce Stress

Scientific studies have shown that correct breathing can help manage stress and stress-related conditions by soothing the autonomic nervous system. Deep breathing can help with a number of disorders, including: Anxiety, Asthma, Chronic Fatigue Syndrome, High Blood Pressure, Insomnia, Pain, Panic Attacks, Eczema and Stress.

When we breathe, the brain sets the breathing rate according to the carbon dioxide levels, rather than the oxygen levels. When a person is under stress, their breathing pattern changes. An anxious person takes small, shallow breaths, using their shoulders rather than their diaphragm to move the air in and out of their lungs. This can prolong feelings of anxiety and cause: Headaches, Fatigue, Insomnia, Chest Tightness and Muscle Aches.

When a person is relaxed, their breathing is slower, more even and gentle. Relaxed breathing seems to calm the nervous system, which can lower blood pressure and heart rate, reduce stress hormones, improve immune system, increase energy, feelings of calm and well-being!

Proper Breathing Helps Control Emotions

Breathing is a necessity of life that usually occurs without much thought. When we are angry, fearful or anxious we tend to over-breathe or breathe too fast! When we experience sadness, suspense, conflict or depression, we tend to under-breathe or hold our breath. These changes are automatic without our deliberate effort to breathe. **When we deliberately think about our breathing we can use it to help control our emotions!**

While the negative emotions cause over-breathing or under-breathing, the positive emotions cause breathing to be deeper, easier and effortless! When we return our breathing to a deep, smooth breathing we can reduce the strength of our negative emotions and restore more peace, serenity and happiness! You can start this process by taking ten deep, smooth, relaxing breaths. With each out breath, say the word "calm" or "relax" silently in your head and there you are relaxing! You have triggered a calming response! This is simple, effective and works!

Start Being Happier & Smile & Laugh More – it's Up to You!

Healthy actions speak louder than words and can elevate your mood if you feel depressed. Take a brisk walk in a natural setting and practice slow, deep breathing – it helps you sort out and solve problems! Spend time with children, it simplifies life and puts everything in perspective. Find the comics in the newspaper or something funny to read and laugh. If someone is upset, try to analyze the situation from that person's perspective. As often as possible make yourself smile and laugh; it opens the blood vessels in the back of your head to physically lift your mood. Choose to be happy in spite of circumstances. No one "makes" you happy – it's an inner attitude that sparkles from within!

Laughter is inner jogging, and good for your body and soul. – Norman Cousins

A laugh is just like sunshine. It freshens up the whole day. – Heart Warmers

Laugh! It puts distance between you and your problems.

Positive affirmations create miracles. – Beatrex Quntanna (Books on amazon.com)

A good laugh is sunshine in a house. – William Makepeace Thackeray

Happiness is a rainbow in your heart – a real health sparkler! – Patricia Bragg

17

Super Power Breathing Calms the Nerves

The greatest tranquilizer for jangled nerves is deep, slow, diaphragmatic breathing. Today's tensions and pressures put additional strain on our nervous systems. The condition is aggravated by poor posture habits and shallow breathing. Your Bragg Super Power Breathing Program will help you correct both of these unhealthy habits . . . while having a calming, healthy effect on your nervous system and entire body!

During your workday, take a minute out of every hour to pause and s-t-r-e-t-c-h from your toes to the top of your head while doing deep, diaphragmatic breathing! Do back and forward shoulder rolls as well! The small amount of time invested in this program will pay dividends in productivity over the course of the day, because you will be able to work faster and with greater efficiency. This is especially important for those restricted to desks, but it's helpful in any kind of work. By oxygenating and relaxing your nerves, you will no longer be distracted or upset by petty annoyances at work or those minor irritations with fellow workers, the boss or friends or family.

Give Thanks to Your Miracle-Working Lungs

Every living thing breathes. Plants breathe through pores in their leaves. In the marvelous balance of Mother Nature, plants breathe in carbon dioxide and give off vital oxygen – while animals inhale oxygen and exhale carbon dioxide. Both thrive in a healthy, natural balance.

Unfortunately humans have played havoc with this natural balance by destroying forests and covering grass with pavement. They continue to poison our already over-burdened air with pollutants from motorized traffic and heavy industry. Wildlife, when it has survived slaughter by man, suffocates in such polluted air. Fish die in polluted waters. How long can people survive in the midst of the environmental poisons which they continually create? This is a question of great concern to us. Read the classic book *Silent Spring* by our friend Rachel Carson, available in libraries or *amazon.com*. If followed, her wise advice would have saved America and nations worldwide billions of dollars! We desperately need more courageous and dedicated people like Rachel Carson to show the world the error of its ways!

The Lower Respiratory System

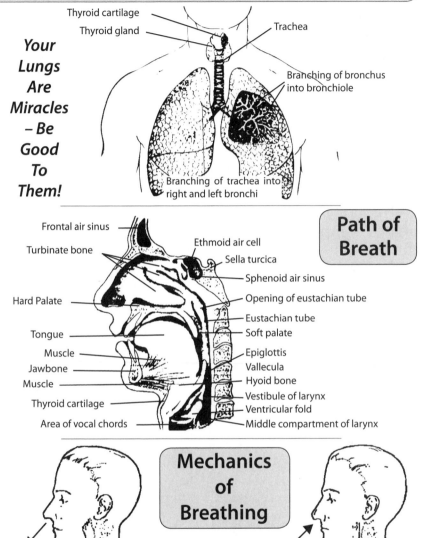

Your Lungs Are Miracles – Be Good To Them!

Thyroid cartilage

Thyroid gland

Trachea

Branching of bronchus into bronchiole

Branching of trachea into right and left bronchi

Path of Breath

Frontal air sinus

Turbinate bone

Hard Palate

Tongue

Muscle

Jawbone

Muscle

Thyroid cartilage

Area of vocal chords

Ethmoid air cell

Sella turcica

Sphenoid air sinus

Opening of eustachian tube

Eustachian tube

Soft palate

Epiglottis

Vallecula

Hyoid bone

Vestibule of larynx

Ventricular fold

Middle compartment of larynx

Mechanics of Breathing

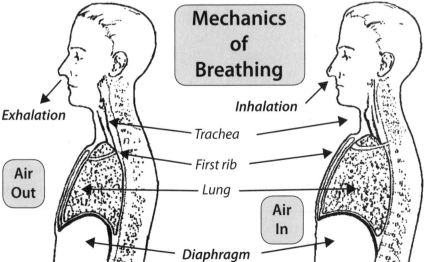

Exhalation

Inhalation

Air Out

Air In

Trachea

First rib

Lung

Diaphragm

Mechanics of Breathing, showing diaphragm position and flexible ribs at exhalation and at inhalation.

19

The Lungs Are Nature's Miracle Breathers

Every animal in the world extracts oxygen from the environment in which it lives. Through their gills, fish extract oxygen from water (H_2O). Insects get oxygen from the air through alveoli or air cells in individual openings set in segments of their bodies. Worms and other invertebrates breathe through the pores of their skin.

Vertebrate animals, and including the human race, have those miracle mechanisms – the lungs. The mechanical equivalent would be a pair of bellows, though the lungs are superior and are far more intricate and adaptable.

Human lungs are a miracle pair of conical-shaped organs composed of spongy, porous tissue. They occupy the thoracic cavity (chest) with the heart in the center, and are protected by the amazingly strong, flexible and resilient rib cage. The apex of each lung reaches just above the collar bone; base extends to the waistline.

What makes up our lungs? About 600 million alveoli – air cells or sacs of elastic tissue – which can expand or contract like tiny balloons. If these little air sacs were flattened out and laid side by side, the flattened alveoli would cover an area of the size of a tennis court. Tiny capillaries (blood vessels) thread elastic walls of each of the millions of air sacs, and it's through these that blood passes to remove its load of carbon dioxide that is expelled as we breathe out and then absorb in vital, life-giving oxygen. The average person has 5 to 6 quarts of blood, which must be continually cleansed.

Air inhaled through the nose and mouth reaches the alveoli through an intricate system of tubes, beginning with the large trachea, or windpipe, which is kept rigid by rings of cartilage in its walls. The trachea extends through the neck into the chest where it divides into two branches (bronchi), each leading into a lung cavity. Each bronchus divides into a number of successively smaller branches to bring air to every air sac. Your lungs are working miracles!

Man is composed of important elements as vital breath,
deeds, thoughts and the senses. – The Upanishads

Success is deciding from the start what end result you want and creating
the circumstances to realize and achieve that result. – Mark Victor Hansen

You Have Lungs – Fill Them Up

Each lung sits perfectly enveloped in a protective elastic membrane, the pleura, whose inner layer is attached to the lung and whose outer layer forms the lining of the thoracic cavity inside the rib cage. One end of each rib is attached to spinal column, but front of the rib cage is open. This allows lungs to expand and contract. When you breathe deeply, filling every air sac, your thoracic cavity expands as lungs breathe in about 500mL. This varies according to body build and size. Lung capacity (the maximum amount of air a person's lungs can hold) is about 4-6 Liters.

This marvelous breathing mechanism is yours for free! You are born with it. It functions without conscious effort, yet without it, you cannot exist! **Start slow, deep relaxed breathing right now. Remember your lungs are miracles!**

Not even the latest medical inventions used by hospitals in emergencies, however ingenious, can equal your human breathing machine! Perhaps if human beings had to pay a fabulous price for their lungs and air, they would use them to full capacity all the time. Think of the big price you pay for only using them partially by shallow breathing. Remember, we are always only one breath away from death!

The Importance of Clean Air to Health

It is essential to breathe clean air – air that's as free as possible from such chemicals as smog, car exhaust, natural gas appliance fumes and many other toxic chemical pollutants. Our air also needs to be as free as possible from dust, dust mites and their fecal matter, animal dander, mold, and pollen. Everyone's health is helped in varying degrees by clean air! It's vitally important to live and work in an area which has clean air and that is free of all harmful fumes! It's also equally important to keep our homes pure, clean and free from clutter, dust and debris! **Most people cannot be truly 100% healthy and well until they breathe clean air, maintain a healthy diet and live a healthy lifestyle!**

Breathing is our connection to life, through the body and heart, leading us to a wholeness of being and giving us spirit for living life to its fullest. – S. Hainer, M.S.

On an average day your faithfully work lungs move enough air in and out to fill a medium-sized room or blow up several thousand party balloons.

Live Longer Breathing Clean Air Deeply

We advise those who live, work, etc. in smog-ridden, polluted cities to obtain a good air filter. We especially recommend filters which contain charcoal and a high efficiency particulate HEPA air filter. The charcoal removes most of the chemicals and the HEPA filter removes most of the particles. To be effective in an average room, the flow rate through the filter should be over 200 cubic feet of air per minute. The wise motorist will also install an air filter in his car for cleaning the air while driving in air-polluted cities. Auto stores and catalogs usually stock them.

When we are born, our lungs are new, fresh, clean, and rosy in color. If we could live in a dust-free atmosphere breathing deeply all our lives, then our lungs would remain *as good as new* for a long, healthy lifetime of use. Yet most people abuse their lungs! Some of this comes from the external causes. The miracle lungs are the only organs of the body which are directly affected by external conditions, specifically, by the air we breathe into them!

Mother Nature has provided protection against a normal amount of dust contamination: tiny hairs in the nose serve as filters and moist mucus in the passages leading to the lungs trap dust particles that we expel through the nose or mouth. The tonsils also serve as guards to trap germs! The lungs protect themselves remarkably well by expelling carbon dioxide through oxygenation and by discharging toxins into the blood for elimination via the kidneys. **Your body is a miracle!**

Unfortunately, most civilized people today live in very unnatural conditions! Almost everywhere there are abnormal amounts of pollutants in the air we breathe, especially in city areas. Our lungs are often overloaded with more contaminants than they can handle! These are passed along into the bloodstream and to other body parts. The lungs of modern city dwellers become brownish from car smog, soot, smoke, etc. Even in most farming areas, the lungs must contend with pollens, excessive dust, poisonous pesticides, fertilizers and other toxic chemicals.

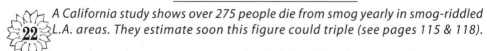

A California study shows over 275 people die from smog yearly in smog-riddled L.A. areas. They estimate soon this figure could triple (see pages 115 & 118).

22

Smoking – A Deadly Habit That Destroys Lungs & Health

With all these nearly inescapable health hazards and growing smog, etc, in the world to overcome, it's incredible that millions of people harm their lungs even more by inhaling deadly tobacco smoke into their lungs daily.

Nicotine is poison! It immediately affects lung function. It constricts your cardiovascular system! It destroys vitamin C, which is vital to your health and immune system! After only 12 hours of not smoking, nicotine blood levels fall and the heart and lungs begin to start healing. If you smoke, please stop now and be loving to your body. (Copy these pages 23-30, and give to smokers.)

The lungs' air sacs are further damaged by tobacco tars and carbon particles. These lodge in the walls of the lungs' important balloon-like cells, causing them to lose their natural elasticity and eventually breaking them down altogether. The result? **Emphysema** – the killer disease in which the destruction of the breathing mechanism is slowly smothering and sadly killing its victim from within!

Of the over 50 million Americans who smoke, one third to one half will die from smoking-related diseases! **Smoking also introduces two deadly poisons into the body: arsenic and carbon monoxide, as well as other toxins.** Compounding these health hazards, smoking creates desire for toxic caffeine and sugar. Moreover, twice as many smokers drink alcohol compared to non-smokers. Smokers have a far greater incidence of cancer of the lungs, larynx, pharynx, esophagus, mouth, colon and breast. **All tobacco products should be banned – they are killers!**

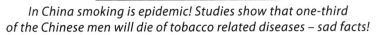

Data from the World Health Organization has found that deaths from lung cancer and chronic obstructive pulmonary disease (COPD) will rise over the next 20 years because of past smoking rates. It describes tobacco smoking as "the most important health hazard" and it maintains that smoking is the main preventable cause of death from lung cancer to coronary artery disease. – bbcnews/health.com

In China smoking is epidemic! Studies show that one-third of the Chinese men will die of tobacco related diseases – sad facts!

Smoking and Your Lungs: What Cigarettes Do

When you smoke cigarettes, many chemicals enter your body through your lungs. Burning tobacco produces more than 4,000 chemicals. Nicotine, carbon monoxide, and tars are some of these substances. Smoking greatly affects your lungs and airways. Smokers get a variety of problems related to breathing. Problems range from an annoying cough to grave illness like tragic emphysema and cancer.

How Your Lungs and Airways Change

Smoking causes many changes in your lungs and airways. Some changes are sudden, last a short time, and then go away. Other changes happen slowly and last a long time, often for the rest of your life. These are chronic changes. **Here's a list of some of the changes that happen in your lungs and airways when you smoke:**

- The cells that produce mucus in your lungs and airways grow. As a result, mucus increases and becomes thicker. Mucus stays in your airways, clogs them, and makes you cough. This extra mucus can easily become infected.

- The lungs have broom-like hairs, called cilia which clean your lungs. A few seconds after you start smoking, the cilia slow down. Smoking one cigarette can slow the action of your cilia for several hours and reduce the number of cilia, so there are fewer cilia to clean your lungs.

- Your lungs and airways get irritated and inflamed. They become narrow and reduce the air flow. Even one or two cigarettes can cause irritation and some coughing.

- When you smoke, your important lungs sadly age faster!!!

- Your lungs can be destroyed – the number of air spaces and blood vessels in the lungs decreases, then less needed oxygen is carried to the rest of your body.

- When you smoke, the natural defenses your lungs have against infection are burdened and do not work well!

- Cigarette smoke has chemicals that can make normal cells change into cancer cells. – *www.upmc.com*

Please visit websites: • *www.cdc.gov/tobacco* • *BeTobaccoFree.hhs.gov*
• *www.lung.org for more info on smoking and damage it does to your lungs!*

E-Cigarettes Are Not Healthy for You!

Electronic cigarettes (or E-Cigs) sales has grown to nearly $3 billion and continues to grow in the U.S. The popularity of these battery-operated nicotine inhalers are all the rage these days; however, much is still unknown about the health risks of E-Cigs or "vaping" as it is often called. What we do know is that it is banned in nearly a dozen countries, and the **World Health Organization is strongly against E-Cigs!**

Yet a recent New Zealand study said tobacco-free E-Cigs have proven as effective as nicotine patches at weaning smokers off their habit. Other specialist have said that E-Cigs has no tar build-up on the lungs as with traditional cigarettes nor are there trace chemicals that come from burning paper or tobacco. But in 2014 Japanese Researchers found harmful carcinogens and formaldehyde were present as well as hazardous chemicals including diethylene glycol, which is found in anti-freeze! Plus, Greek researchers found *E-Cigs increased breathing difficulty, and other studies have suggested that secondhand vapor poses health risks! The American Lung Association and other authorities assert that they are NOT safer than regular cigarettes!*

E-Cigs "Nicotine" Worse Than Cigarettes

Instead of burning tobacco, E-Cigs are battery powered devices that heat up flavored, nicotine-laced liquid. This "liquid nicotine" is extracted from tobacco and tinctured with a cocktail of flavorings, colorings and chemicals like formaldehyde and propylene glycol. **Scientist say E-Cigs contain 10 times as many cancer chemicals as cigarettes.** Even in tiny amounts, ingested or absorbed through the skin, can cause vomiting, seizures and can even be lethal! In one year the accidental poisoning cases linked to e-liquids jumped 300%. **The nicotine inside E-cartridges is very addictive.** When you stop using it, you can get withdrawal symptoms including feeling irritable, depressed, restless and anxious.

Your lungs are precious and needed every minute of your life. It's important to keep them clean & away from all smoke! – Patricia Bragg, ND, PhD.

All Tobacco & Nicotine Should Be Banned – it's a Killer!
Shocking Sad Facts: Children and teenagers make up 90% of all the new smokers in United States. Sadly teenage and college smoking is on rise!

E-Cigarettes, Young Adults and Tobacco

A study found nearly 1.8 million young people have tried E-Cigarettes and the number of kids in grades 6-12 who have tried electronic cigarettes tripled from 2011 to 2014, according to Center for Disease Control. One of the major claims in popularizing E-Cigs is their (false) harmlessness as compared to regular cigarettes. Now, researchers are revealing how bad they actually are! Nicotine is an addictive chemical and E-Cigs could be leading kids to use tobacco. **The candy and fruit flavors added to E-Cigs are geared to make them popular among younger generation.** Once addicted to nicotine, users move on to using tobacco with all the health risks! Our recommendation is to treat E-Cigs the same way as conventional cigarettes – STOP SMOKING! These are "gateway" habits that can lead to harder drugs and other very dangerous activities! Over 60% of the children who smoke pot before the age of 15 move into the deadly drugs: cocaine, heroin, hallucinogens, etc.

Stop Smoking – Save Your Lungs and Life

In our Bragg Health Crusade Lectures throughout the world, we have had thousands of health students who were smokers; some for as long as 40 years. We inspired them to stop smoking and take charge of their health! You can too! Smokers should read about deadly effects of smoking to the heart and overall health in book, *Healthy Heart: Keep Your Cardiovascular System Healthy and Fit at Any Age (pgs. 237-239)*.

Here's a tip from a writer friend of ours who, over the years, had acquired the habit of lighting a cigarette whenever she paused to compose her next sequence of thoughts. She said, "When it dawned on me what I was doing, I felt like a complete fool. I stopped smoking! It was destroying my health and slowly killing me. Now, instead of a cigarette, I take a full, deep breath and I'm healthier and my thoughts come faster and more clearly than ever!"

She finally realized that she did this because her brain was calling for more oxygen! What she actually needed and wanted was a deep breath – but she was inhaling smoke instead of life-giving oxygen, thus defeating her purpose.

One Exception: *A special blend of marijuana, for medicinal purposes, relieves pain in adults and stops seizures in children.* – Dr. Sanjay Gupta see video: DrMercola.com

If you are a smoker, try this! When you want to smoke a cigarette or cigar or pipe – stop! Instead, take a long, slow, deep breath – filling every air sac in your lungs – and hold it, allowing your red blood cells to become more oxygenated – then exhale slowly and completely. Empty every bit of poison from your lungs. You will feel a new surge of energy from the top of your scalp to the soles of your feet! It's a relaxing and incredibly rejuvenating sensation which you can never get from using tobacco or any other artificial stimulant! The surest way to quit a bad habit is to replace it with a good one!!! Start today to make the effort to stop as a positive step towards living The Bragg Healthy Lifestyle!

TO ALL SMOKERS:

The greatest benefit to your life and health would be to replace deadly smoking with healthy deep breathing!

Wise Teens Talk About Stopping Smoking

Ex-smoking teens testify that their life is better, self-esteem higher and hope and joy for the future more profound after they quit smoking! Often these misguided, unfortunate children begin smoking before they are old enough to appreciate their hard-working lungs! They begin filling their miracle breathing lungs with health destroying tobacco, some when they are 16, 14 and even 10 years old! Stan B. recalls, "I started smoking when I was 12, to look cool." Susan W. says, "I smoked 2 packs a day from the time I was 16."

As horrifying as these shocking stories are, we can take heart from these youngsters and learn a lesson from their resiliency. Though they are young and the challenge they face is difficult, many teen smokers are winning the battle against smoking habit, and feeling healthier and happier as a result! Bragg Health Foundation is helping, (pages iii-v). When it comes to quitting, Stan B. says, "It's not easy, I look at my parents who've smoked for 25 years! I know I don't want to be sucking smoke into my lungs and coughing like them."

Adults and children from poor households are employed in tobacco farming. They are vulnerable to "green tobacco sickness", caused by the nicotine absorbed through the skin from handling wet tobacco leaves. – World Health Organization

---

The global tobacco epidemic, if unchecked will kill one billion people in the 21st century. – ASH.org

Every smoking teen should remember that they are not alone in the struggle to quit, and that their goal is within reach. Many young adults now choose a healthy quality of life over one of the greatest destroyers of our time – smoking! And, should any smoking teen find themselves wavering in their efforts to quit, they should remember the words of ex-smoking teen Ann S., who explains, "The biggest reward was that my self-esteem became so much better – I don't need a cigarette to make everything okay. I have made positive changes, enjoy a healthy lifestyle and have more money, time and energy!"

Quit Smoking – See the Difference it Makes!

• **20 MINUTES AFTER QUITTING:** Your blood pressure and pulse rate drop to normal. The temperature of your hands and feet increases to normal.

• **8 HOURS AFTER QUITTING:** The carbon monoxide level in your blood drops to normal. Amazingly, the life-giving oxygen level in your blood then increases to normal.

• **24 HOURS AFTER QUITTING:** You substantially lessen your chances of having a heart attack or stroke.

• **48 HOURS AFTER QUITTING:** Your nerve endings start regrowing and your ability to taste and smell is enhanced.

• **2 WEEKS TO 3 MONTHS AFTER QUITTING:** Your circulation improves. Brisk walking and exercise becomes easier. Your lung function increases and improves as much as 30 percent.

• **1 TO 9 MONTHS AFTER QUITTING:** Coughing, sinus congestion, fatigue and shortness of breath decreases. Your lungs and body are becoming cleaner and more resistant to infection.

• **1 YEAR AFTER QUITTING:** Excess risk for coronary heart disease decreases to an amazing 50% that of a smoker's.

• **2 TO 3 YEARS AFTER QUITTING:** The risk for coronary heart disease and stroke decrease compared to those of people who have never smoked. Also less chance of osteoporosis.

• **5 YEARS AFTER QUITTING:** Lung cancer death rate for the former one-pack-per-day smoker decreases by over half. Risks of mouth and throat cancer are half those of smokers.

• **10 TO 15 YEARS AFTER QUITTING:** Lung cancer death rate is almost that of non-smokers. Pre-cancerous cells are replaced. Risks for mouth, throat, esophagus, bladder, kidney, breast and pancreas cancer decrease. – *Prevention Magazine*

More than 40 million Americans are cigarette smokers. Nearly 70% of smokers report they want to quit, more than 42% say they've tried to quit during the past year (there was only a 10% decrease in cigarette sales in U.S.) – CDC

Deadly Smoking – A Health Hazard to Avoid – What it Does to You and Those Around You!

When people inhale deadly tobacco smoke into their miracle lungs, the protective cilia hairs filter out much of the smoke's harmful substances before it is exhaled. This means that while harmful toxins are trapped in the delicate linings of the smokers' lungs, fewer of these toxins are re-released into the air for others to breathe in. However, between a smoker's deadly puffs, the cigarette burns directly into the air. This smoke is known as "secondhand, side-stream" smoke, but it should be called "direct" smoke. Smoke that burns directly into the air is completely unfiltered and more deadly than the smokers' smoke! **Stay away from all deadly smoke!**

Recent studies establish that people who live or work around smokers are more likely to develop lung and sinus damage than smokers! For asthma or bronchitis sufferers, this exposure is very damaging. In addition to these dangers, "direct" smoke irritates the eyes, nose and throat and smells up everything it touches (rooms, hotels, offices, carpets, drapes, cars and everything around smoking).

For the cigarette smoker, whose miracle lungs have unfortunately become the filters protecting the body from the deadly smoke, the effects are equally – if not more – damaging. Tar begins to collect in the lungs once there is too much to be removed through the lungs' normal cleaning processes. This means the over-burdened lungs can no longer clean normal contaminants they have to deal with. Dirt inhaled into the alveoli – which is normally trapped in a layer of sticky mucus and carried out of the lungs by the wavelike motions of the tiny cilia hairs – becomes trapped and stuck in the lungs! The cilia hairs become paralyzed by tar, so the normal cleansing (drain) procedures break down and the airways become clogged. This makes the lungs resort to coughing, spitting and respiratory – breathing attacks, flu, etc. in an effort to expel the contaminated, clogging toxins, tar and mucus.

There is good news. When a person stops smoking the cilia hairs begin to heal and move again. Smokers – stop now, you begin cleansing and healing immediately!

Smoking cigarettes is know to cause damage to every organ in your body. – CDC

DEADLY SMOKING FACTS!

- Tobacco use and also second-hand smoke will eventually kill over one fifth of world population – now 6 million yearly.

- Of the over 50 million Americans who smoke, one third to one half will die from a smoke-related disease and all will reduce their life expectancy by an average of nine years.

- Smoking acts as either a stimulant or a depressant – depending upon the smoker's emotional state at the time.

- The average pack-a-day smoker takes about 70,000 *hits* of deadly nicotine each year. Do visit and read: *www.ash.org*

- "Second hand smoke" hurts non-smokers: it speeds up their heart rate, raises blood pressure and doubles the amount of deadly carbon monoxide in their blood. It's a killer!

- Secondary deadly smoke contains more nicotine, tar and cadmium than mainstream smoke (leads to hypertension, emphysema, cancer, and asthma) and is killing millions!

- Babies born to mothers who smoke tend to have lower body weight, smaller lungs, poor health and many develop asthma.

- Lung illnesses are twice as common in smokers' children.

- Children and teenagers make up 90% of the new smokers in the United States – and teenage (deadly) smoking is on the rise!

- The death rate from breast cancer ranges from 25% to 75% higher among women who smoke. *www.BreastCancer.org*

- Female smokers may face a higher risk of lung cancer – as much as twice the risk of male smokers, according to a study done by Dr. Harvey Risch at Yale University.

- For both men and women, those who smoked more than two packs a day were 50 times more likely to develop lung cancer than those who never smoked (*National Cancer Institute*).

- Your body contains almost 100,000 miles of blood vessels. Smoking ages and constricts those vessels, depriving your body of important, rich oxygen it needs, lack causes serious illness.

- Tobacco is the main introduction to more deadly drugs!!!

- Teens who smoke are far more likely to engage in other risky and life-threatening behaviors (including using other dangerous drugs; violence; hatred; gang involvement; carrying weapons; and engaging in premarital sex which often results in pregnancy or disease) than non-smoking healthy teens.

- Cataracts, cancer, angina, arteriosclerosis, osteoporosis, chronic bronchitis, asthma, high blood pressure, impotency and respiratory ailments are linked to all forms of smoking.

30

QUIT SMOKING! All smokers must stop this vicious, deadly smoking habit that destroys health, youth, energy and life!

Chapter 5

Common Cold – The Body's Miracle Cleansing Process

Any one day in winter, over 30 million Americans suffer with a bad cold. Adults average five to six colds per season, while children and teenagers often get double that amount. The body wants the toxins and mucus out!

Are these colds necessary? How do people *catch cold?* What causes the common cold? Medical Science has learned how to control many diseases that are far more serious, but remains baffled by the common cold. Is the culprit an unfiltered virus? Is it brought on by sitting in a draft, getting chilled, or getting one's feet wet, as is often suggested by mothers through the ages?

Colds Clean Out Mucus and Toxins

While the theories are many, there seems to be only one sure fact – people who are in perfect health don't *catch colds.* My dad spent a year living in the Arctic among the Eskimos. He never had a cold, and neither did they. He had the same experience in the South Seas, in the Balkans, among the nomads of the Middle East and with the native tribes of Africa. The common factor among all these people is that they breathe pure air, eat simple natural foods and get plenty of exercise and sleep. By following this same basic healthy lifestyle, my Dad remained free of colds even in the midst of civilization.

Based on his research, he found that the *common cold* is Mother Nature's and God's method of detoxifying the body. Most people are shallow breathers. And most live on an unhealthy diet of devitalized foods. Toxins start accumulating and clogging their bodies. That's why it's important to live a healthy lifestyle, plus some fasting.

"When you feel a cold or any illness coming on, or are just depressed – it is best to fast! Each time you fast, you will feel better. Your body will then have a chance to cleanse and heal and rebuild its immune system by regular fasting. Bragg Health Books were my conversion to the healthy way. Everyone should read Bragg's "Miracle of Fasting" book!" (see pages 237-239)
– James Balch, M.D., Co-Author, "Prescription for Nutritional Healing"

The Body Self-Cleanses, Repairs & Heals

When toxicity of accumulated poisons, mucus, etc., exceeds the body's tolerance, natural vital forces set up a miracle *cleansing-healing* (common colds) crisis. The body induces rise in body temperature (fever) to burn up the many toxins, while others are eliminated by heavy discharge of mucus from nose, mouth and throat. If the toxic overload is heavy, there may be discharge of mucus from bowels and perhaps diarrhea.

Instead of being alarmed, be grateful your body's natural Vital Forces are strong enough to take command by pushing out the toxins you have accumulated! Don't try to block this natural detox and healing process with antibiotics, aspirin, etc. Work with Mother Nature. Breathe deeply and fully to supply your body with the great purifier: oxygen. Rest and fast (page 146). Do a distilled water fast (8 glasses daily) or try fresh juice fast (page 144). It's best to take only liquids during this cleansing and healing crisis. Your body will fight for its life against a great deal of abuse. When you follow Mother Nature's and God's Laws and live Bragg Healthy Lifestyle you can create a painless, tireless and ageless body. Miracles can happen!

Colds and Oxygen are Great Cleansers

If you *catch cold,* remember you're going through a detox, natural cleansing and healing crisis. Heed the warning – fast! Mother Nature is telling you: *"You have allowed your body to become polluted with toxic wastes and maybe by overeating. Work with me now by fasting – to cleanse your body of these toxins. Once this cleansing crisis has passed, now keep your body clean by following my Laws of Natural Living!"*

Often people tell us that they have a bad case of the *flu.* When we ask where they got it, this is what we hear – *"The flu's going around. Everyone's got it."* We then ask, *"Where can we find it? We'd like to meet some flu germs!"* They stare at us in utter amazement. To help them out of their mental confusion, we explain that when you breathe fully, live a healthy lifestyle and eat natural foods, free from all refining, processing and chemical additives – it's then that you can build a powerful immunity against germs, viruses and illness!

The body is self-cleansing and self-healing when you give it a chance with a **32** *fasting detox cleanse and living a healthy lifestyle!* – Patricia Bragg, ND, PhD.

Oxygen Cleanses and Nourishes

No germ can live in freshly squeezed organic orange juice because there is nothing in pure orange juice for it to feed on. All germs, regardless of their names, are scavengers! They feed on toxic decaying matter.

It's our personal opinion, based on experience and research, that a 100% healthy, natural foods diet – in combination with the enormous amount of pure oxygen pumped into the body by the vigorous breathing exercises taught in this book will help provide a natural immunity against most infectious diseases and germs.

Oxygen is not only the energizing factor which makes it possible for the body to eliminate putrefied matter on which germs thrive, it helps exterminate germs! As you deeply breathe more oxygen into your body and nourish it with organic, healthy foods, you give your body a greater ability to ward off germs and infections!

When we practice Super Power Breathing, we increase our cardiovascular respiratory power! We purify and energize our bloodstream to carry more powerful, revitalizing oxygen to the heart and entire cardiovascular system. Start practicing today – you will benefit greatly.

Oil of Oregano Nature's Versatile Healer & Detox

Oil of Oregano: *is a powerful herbal body defender and cleanser and is used to fight: viruses; flus; colds; allergies; asthma; E. coli; Salmonella; parasitic yeast and bacterial infections; upset stomach; menstrual problems; urinary tract problems and arthritis. Take with food. Available in caps or drops at Health and Vitamin Stores. (When needed for winter cold maintenance use caps and drops, and do the Breathing Detox below.)* – Patricia Bragg

Helpful Breathing Detox: *Place 2-3 drops of "Oil of Oregano" in 2 quarts boiling water. Put towel over head, breathe in vapors through mouth, then nose. It's powerful, close eyes! This opens up lungs to remove congestion. Relieves colds, flu, bronchitis congestion. Do as needed 1-3x daily. Also try nasal wash (page 37) or add 1 drop oil in juice or ACV drink (page 149).*

Breathe Deep Yogi Organic Tea *helps clear breathing passages and nourishes lung tissues. This healing formula utilizes licorice, basil, cinnamon, peppermint, ginger and herb thyme to loosen phlegm and relax muscles of respiratory tract.*

A healthy body is a guest-chamber for the soul; a sick body is a prison.

Improved lung function guards against onset of illness. – Holger Schunemann, MD

THE MIRACLES OF APPLE CIDER VINEGAR FOR A STRONGER, LONGER, HEALTHIER LIFE

> **The old adage is true:**
> *"An apple a day keeps the doctor away."*

- Helps promote a youthful skin and vibrant healthy body
- Helps remove artery plaque, infections and body toxins
- Helps fight germs, viruses, bacteria and mold naturally
- Helps retard old age onset in humans, pets and farm animals
- Helps regulate calcium metabolism
- Helps keep blood the right consistency
- Helps regulate women's menstruation, relieves PMS, and UTI
- Helps normalize urine pH, relieving frequent urge to urinate
- Helps digestion, assimilation and helps balance the pH
- Helps protect against food poisoning and even brings relief if you do get it
- Helps relieve sore throats, laryngitis and throat tickles and cleans out throat and gum toxins
- Helps detox the body so sinus, asthma and flu sufferers can breathe easier and more normally
- Helps banish acne, athlete's foot, soothes burns, sunburns
- Helps prevent itching scalp, baldness, and dry hair
- Helps banish dandruff, rashes, and shingles
- Helps fight arthritis and helps remove crystals and toxins from joints, tissues, organs and entire body
- Helps control and normalize body weight

– Paul C. Bragg, ND, PhD., Health Crusader, Originator of Health Stores

Our sincere blessings to you, dear friends, who make our lives so worthwhile and fulfilled by reading our teachings on natural living as our Creator laid down for us to follow. He wants us to follow the simple path of natural living. This is what we teach in our books and health crusades worldwide. Our prayers reach out to you and your loved ones for the best in health and happiness. We must follow the laws He has laid down for us, so we can reap this precious health physically, mentally, emotionally and spiritually!

HAVE AN APPLE HEALTHY LIFE!

With Love,

Braggs Organic Raw Unfiltered Apple Cider Vinegar with the "Mother Enzyme" is #1 food I recommend to stop heartburn, gerds, gas, indigestion and for maintaining body's vital acid-alkaline balance and digestion.
– Gabriel Cousens, M.D., Author, "Conscious Eating"

Chapter 6

Your Miracle Nose – Pathway to the Lungs

The Bragg Super Power Breathing technique is the most essential part of The Bragg Healthy Lifestyle. Your nose and nasal passageways are essential factors in all your breathing. So it's important that we understand the nose and the vital health role it plays in breathing.

The nose is a system of passages and hollow spaces that link the external nose to the eyes, ears, mouth and throat. It is through this intricate pathway that oxygen-rich air travels from our nose to our lungs. You might wonder why we have all this complicated breathing mechanism made up of cartilage, bone, and soft tissue organized into several pairs of hollow air-spaces called sinuses. When afflicted with some sinus or nasal complaint you might think it just can't be worth all the trouble. After all, the mouth and throat seem to do the breathing work just fine – and it's just a simple and direct air pathway to the lungs.

We Mostly Breathe Through the Nose

We do most breathing through the nose. That means that the oxygen required to nourish our bodies moves through the nose 22,000 or more times a day, depending upon whether you are a shallow, deep or slow breather. So then, why is this part of our body so complex and a site of so many health complaints? The answer is that the nose is a lot more than just a pathway for air to get to the lungs, it's a miracle-working part of your body!

Shallow breathing helps to increase symptoms of almost every known sickness!

The quality of the blood depends largely upon its oxygenation in the lungs.
– Basic Physiology

Your nose is the only organ able to properly prepare the air you breathe. Mouth breathing and resultant over-breathing elevates your blood pressure and heart rate and worsens asthma, allergies, rhinitis, sleep apnea, and deprives your heart, brain and other organs of optimal oxygenation. – Breathing.com

Your Nose is a Miracle Air-Filtration System

The hollow spaces of the nose – called sinuses – act as "echo chambers" (eight *air pockets*), which make our voices resonate (unless sinuses are stuffed up). These open spaces (located behind our eyebrows, nose, cheeks, and between the eyes) also give us better balance and cushion the brain from blows to the head. Our sense of smell is located in the nose. The most important function of the nose, the sinuses and nose hairs, is to condition and filter the air as it passes through to your faithful, hard-working lungs.

The membranes of the nose and sinuses produce between a pint and a quart of mucus every day. These secretions line the walls of the nose and sinuses and are always on the move. As the mucus passes through the sinus cavities, it collects dust particles, bacteria and other air pollutants that were breathed in along with the oxygen-rich air that nourishes every corner of the body. These same airways are lined with little filter hairs (called *cilia*) which strongly try to keep out all dust and pollutants from the air we breathe.

As you can see, God entrusts some very important duties to the nose. It's the nose that tries its best to protect the lungs and all your body cells from any airborne pollutants and contaminants! Under healthy conditions, our lungs receive clean air even with some pollution, thanks to our nose filters! Sadly, in the world many areas have heavy pollution that plagues our air and takes its toll on the health of the body! The nose takes the brunt of the attack, then lungs and the body.

Sinusitis Causes Breathing & Infection Problems

Sinus complaints usually are signs of the nose trying to do its job of protecting the lungs in troubled times. The nasal passages can suffer from the contaminants they work hard to block. Sometimes the sinuses become irritated or inflamed from air pollution, smoke, mold, pet dander, infection, or an allergy attack (for most common food allergies see page 40) brought on by some of these irritating toxic factors (*nasal wash helps heal see next page*).

A large percent of sinus problems are caused by bacteria, pollutants, such as smoke and dust, allergies and overuse of nasal decongestant medication.

Blocked Sinuses Breed Health Problems

When nose and sinuses become over-burdened, they secrete mucus and swell. This blocks the openings and prevents flow of mucus and air. This causes a breathing problem that creates an environment where bacteria can flourish. This unhealthy situation weakens the nose and sets stage for sinus and asthma problems, poor breathing and infections, etc.

Many people who suffer from blocked and painful sinuses run to drug store for over-the-counter medical relief. They hope nasal sprays will relieve their breathing problems. Many don't follow directions and abuse the sprays, often becoming addicted with disastrous consequences. Forcing sinuses open continually can cause harm, because they close up to protect lungs from airborne toxins, etc. "If your sinuses are the problem, longer use puts you at risk for a chronic situation of diminishing returns," says Joel Saper, MD. Instead of quick-fix relief of a drug, take a long-term view of your nose's health. Remember, your nose is the pathway to your lungs, and the point of entry for the body's most needed, elemental nutrient – oxygen. Your nose deserves to be treated with loving, gentle care!

Nasal Wash Brings Relief & Healing

Nasal spray abuse can also cause a secondary illness, *rhinitis medicamentosa,* when the nose becomes inflamed by the medicine itself. In addition to healthy living and avoiding all dairy, you can relieve sinusitis symptoms and bolster your nose health with this simple nasal wash.

Simple Apple Cider Vinegar Nasal Wash

To help relieve nasal mucus symptoms naturally and safely, do simple Apple Cider Vinegar Nasal (sniff) Wash. Add 1/2 tsp. Bragg ACV to one cup warm distilled water. Cup in hand, sniff up left nostril, roll head back, then side to side, lean over bowl, blow out mucus. Then repeat with other nostril, do 3 times. Do 2-3 times daily until mucus conditions subside. Also enjoy Bragg Apple Cider Vinegar Health Drink 3 times daily (see recipe on page 149).

BRONCHIAL DRAINAGE: *Use gravity to move secretions (mucus, etc.) from small airways into larger ones & out for easier breathing. All positions are done with head lower than hips on a slant or ironing board. You can try laying on your back, stomach & sides. Try each position 5-15 minutes.*

Other Healthy Ways to Unblock Your Sinuses

Herbs (tea or cap): fenugreek, echinacea, anise, marshmallow and red clover, help to loosen phlegm and clear congestion; rosehips, horehound and mullein help relieve symptoms. Golden Seal an anti-microbial and immune booster herb is also beneficial for respiratory conditions. Ginger another herb you can use by steeping thin slices in hot water for 10 minutes, then drink it as tea. Inhaling warm vapors can also relieve pain and pressure.

Neti Pots: treat congested sinuses, colds and allergies. Use to rinse nasal passages with saline (salt-based) solution. Make sure to use only distilled or sterilized water – DO NOT use tap water! Find Neti pots at pharmacies, health food stores and online.

Inhale eucalyptus, lavender, peppermint or basil oils: put few drops in boiling water, turn heat off, carefully breathe vapors.

Drink 8 or more glasses distilled water daily: You can add Bragg Organic Vinegar to 3 of them – recipe page 149.

Solve Sinus and Allergy Problems

For a healthy nose, it's essential you live The Bragg Healthy Lifestyle. A balanced, healthy life is the basis for good health! A healthy, happy head and body are necessary preconditions to a healthy nose. If you live in a polluted area, smokers, etc. or if sinuses are already damaged from the hard work of protecting your lungs, buy a high-efficiency HEPA (microscopic pores remove almost all particles) air filtration system. This pre-filters and cleans the air you breathe, making the job easier for your nose. Also enjoy herbal teas (see above) or take them in capsule form. You must be intelligent about allergies. If you know you're allergic to particular substances, take precautions to avoid them. If you suspect allergies, take all necessary steps to learn if and what you are allergic to (do test next page). The most common allergens are mold spores, animal dandruff, and house dust. Also, food allergies (see chart next page) are high sources of allergic reactions; they are associated with the nose, sinus, and mucus complaints.

Apple Cider Vinegar Cayenne Pepper Cold Remedy

Soothe That Sinus Pain with Bragg Raw Apple Cider Vinegar Brew: *Try out this strange and spicy brew and find some relief! 4 Tbsps. each of water and Bragg Apple Cider Vinegar, 1 Tbsp. honey, 1 tsp cayenne pepper and 1 wedge lemon. Bring water to boil. Combine water and ACV in a small glass or mug. Add honey and cayenne pepper. Stir well. Add squeeze of lemon. Start drinking.*

It is of utmost importance to avoid dairy products. Millions suffer allergic reactions (mucus, colds, etc.) to dairy products because they are very unhealthy for the nose and the whole body. Dairy proteins can cause the nose and throat airway passages to swell. They also produce mucus-causing sinus discomfort and bacterial mucus conditions. If you snore (page 99) or suffer a sinus problem, a non-dairy diet brings miracle improvements!

Read 2 important books on milk and why best to avoid:

- *Mad Cows and Milk Gate* by Virgil Hulse M.D.
  - *Milk, the Deadly Poison* by Robert Cohen

Both books on *amazon.com*. Also visit these websites:
- *www.notmilk.com* • *www.strongbones.org*
- *pcrm.org* (Physicians Committee for Responsible Medicine)

Allergies, Daily Journal & Dr. Coca's Pulse Test

Almost every known food may cause some allergic reaction at times. Thus, foods used in *elimination diets* may cause allergic reactions in some individuals. Some are listed among the **Most Common Food Allergies** (see next page). Since reaction to these foods is generally low, they are widely used in making test diets. By keeping a food journal and tracking your pulse rate after meals you will soon know your problem foods. Allergic foods cause pulse rate to go up. (Take base pulse, for 1 minute, before meals, then 30 minutes after meals, and also before bed. If it increases 8-10 beats per minute – check foods for allergies.)

A Self-Test for Food Allergy Problems

Do a 3-day fast on distilled water and most of your food allergies will clear up. Record in Daily Journal (page 151) and then allow your usual foods back into your diet, one at a time. Soon you will discover which allergy foods to eliminate from your diet that cause problems.

The body is self-cleansing and self-healing! It is our duty if we want vibrant, glorious health, to do all we can to make the body work efficiently to maintain vital, super health. Not only is a healthy diet necessary, but so are good sleeping habits, outdoor physical activity, full, deep breathing and a serene, peaceful mind. We cannot live by bread alone. We must have spiritual food. And also strive for a perfect healthy balance: physical, mental, emotional and spiritual!

If your body has a reaction after eating some particular food, especially if it happens each time you eat that food, you may have an allergy. Some allergic reactions are: wheezing, sneezing, stuffy nose, nasal drip or mucus, dark circles, eye watering or waterbags under eyes, headaches, feeling light-headed or dizzy, fast heart beat, stomach or chest pains, diarrhea, extreme thirst, breaking out in a rash, swelling of extremities or stomach bloating, etc. (Do read Dr. Arthur Coca's book, *The Pulse Test* – available on *www.amazon.com*)

If you know what you're allergic to, you are lucky; if you don't, you had better find out as fast as possible and eliminate all irritating foods from your diet. To re-evaluate your daily life and have a health guide to your future, start a daily journal (8½ x 11 notebook page 151) of foods eaten, your pulse rate before and after meals and your reactions, moods, energy levels, weight, elimination and sleep patterns. You will discover the foods and situations causing problems. By charting your diet you will be amazed at the effects of eating certain foods. We have kept daily journals for years.

If you are hypersensitive to certain foods, you must omit them from your diet! There are hundreds of allergies and of course it's impossible here to take up each one. Many have allergies to milk, wheat, or some are allergic to all grains. Visit web: *FoodAllergy.org*. Your daily journal will help you discover and accurately pinpoint the foods and situations causing you problems. Start your journal today!

Most Common Food Allergies

- *MILK: Butter, Cheese, Cottage Cheese, Ice Cream, Milk, Yogurt*
- *CEREALS & GRAINS: Wheat, Corn, Buckwheat, Oats, Rye*
- *EGGS: Cakes, Custards, Dressings, Mayonnaise, Noodles*
- *FISH: Shellfish, Crabs, Lobster, Shrimp, Shadroe*
- *MEATS: Bacon, Chicken, Pork, Sausage, Veal, Smoked Products*
- *FRUITS: Citrus Fruits, Melons, Strawberries*
- *NUTS: Peanuts, Pecans, Walnuts, chemically dried, preserved Nuts*
- *MISCELLANEOUS: Chocolate, China Black Tea, Cocoa, Coffee, MSG, Palm and Cottonseed Oils, Salt, Spices and allergic reactions often caused by toxic pesticides on salad greens, vegetables, fruits, etc.*

What a person eats becomes his own body chemistry.
– Paul C. Bragg, ND, PhD., Originator of Health Stores

Take Precautions to Prevent Nosebleeds

Another common health complaint is nosebleeds. Various conditions cause nosebleeds, including blows to face, excessive dryness, changes in atmospheric pressure, and scratching or blowing the nose too strenuously.

Nosebleeds can be classified either as anterior (discharging out the nose) or posterior (discharging down the throat). Posterior bleeding originates in the sinus cavities behind eyebrows, nose or between eyes. No matter what position the person is in, blood will drain out the back of the mouth and down the throat. This condition can affect the elderly that have high blood pressure and they need their doctor's advice. The anterior nosebleed is common variety and flows out nostrils – although if one lies down, the blood may flow down throat. Rarely serious, it can usually be treated by applying pressure to the nose and ice to the injured area. (Soak cotton ball in Bragg Apple Cider Vinegar, lightly pack in the nostril and press – this can help blood to coagulate.)

Because excessively dry air can cause nasal membranes to crack, form crusts and bleed, increase the humidity in your house if you reside in a dry climate. You can do this with a commercial humidifier. If you need a quick fix, place a pan of boiling water in a small room. To help alleviate dry, sore nasal membranes, nightly gently pat aloe-vera, vitamin E, Bragg Organic Olive Oil or comfrey ointment inside your nose.

Nosebleeds might be caused by a vitamin K deficiency. This is a crucial mineral for normal blood clotting. If you don't have your fair share, your nose will be more likely to bleed at the least provocation. You can remedy this situation by practicing wise, healthy, natural eating habits. Best vitamin K sources include sprouts, all dark-green leafy vegetables, sea greens, oats, eggs, molasses, alfalfa, wheatgrass, barley and spirulina, etc.

Vitamin K helps to prevent hardening of the arteries, which is a common factor in coronary disease and heart failure. Research suggests vitamin K may help to keep calcium out of your artery linings and other body tissues, where it can cause damage. The latest studies show Vitamin K with vitamin D, prevents calcification in your coronary arteries, thereby preventing heart disease. – DrMercola.com

Take Time for 12 Things

1. Take time to **Work** –
    it is the price of success.
2. Take time to **Think** –
    it is the source of power.
3. Take time to **Play** –
    it is the secret of youth.
4. Take time to **Read** –
    it is the foundation of knowledge.
5. Take time to **Worship** –
    it is the highway of reverence and
    washes the dust of earth from our eyes.
6. Take time to **Help and Enjoy Friends** –
    it is the source of happiness.
7. Take time to **Love and Share** –
    it is the one sacrament of life.
8. Take time to **Dream** –
    it hitches the soul to the stars.
9. Take time to **Laugh** –
    it is the singing that helps life's loads.
10. Take time for **Beauty** –
    it is everywhere in nature.
11. Take time for **Health** –
    it is the true wealth and treasure of life.
12. Take time to **Plan** –
    it is the secret of being able to have time
    for the first 11 things.

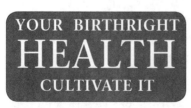

YOUR BIRTHRIGHT
HEALTH
CULTIVATE IT

**Have an
Apple
Healthy Life!**
3 John 2

*Teach me Thy way O Lord, and
lead me in a simple plain path.* – Psalm 27:11

Chapter 7

Your Diaphragm – The Key to Bragg Super Power Breathing

What is our secret of deep Super Power Breathing? How can you draw air into the very base of your lungs? Not by merely sniffing it in through your nose nor by gasping it in through your mouth!

Babies breathe naturally by using their diaphragms to create suction which pulls air into the lungs. Air may enter the body through either the nose or the mouth. But the pulling force which draws the air in, filling the air sacs of the lungs to capacity, comes from the strong muscular action of the powerful diaphragm.

The miracle diaphragm is a dome-shaped sheet of strong muscle fibers. It separates the thoracic (upper) half of your body, which contains the heart and lungs – from the abdominal (lower) cavity, which houses the organs of digestion and elimination. The diaphragm stretches from the sternum (breastbone) in front and across the bottom of the ribs to the backbone.

As the diaphragm expands and flattens, it then moves downward, producing suction within the chest cavity and pulling air into the lungs (inhalation). When the diaphragm relaxes and rises, it forces air out of the lungs (exhalation). Both operations are equally important: inhalation to bring in life-giving oxygen; exhalation to expel all of the collected poisonous carbon dioxide.

Before you can take a deep breath, you have to give one away. Why? Because, when you've been breathing in a shallow manner (from your chest), if you try and take a deep inhale, you just can't do it. All you can do is take a more labored, shallow breath from your chest. Slow, deep breathing out, and then breathing in, a full deep breath – works miracles! – See web: AnxietyCoach.com

During times of stress and anger, we tend to inhale and hold our breath. The most significant, therapeutic aspect of diaphragmatic breathing is the exhalation – which is best at least two times the length of the inhalation. The slow exhalation alerts the body that it can relax and resume essential body functions and not remain in state of upset, fight or flight. – Paul C. Bragg

Diaphragmatic Versus Chest Breathing

Chest breathing results from the movement of the rib section of the trunk, especially the upper section of the chest. When a person inhales, the chest expands, becoming larger. When he exhales, the chest relaxes, and then becomes smaller. When performed to the limit of inhalation and exhalation, it's an excellent form of internal exercise that helps the whole waist and internal organs. It also develops the chest and has many other health benefits.

A great deal is made about *chest expansion . . .* the number of inches which the chest expands from a relaxed position (after exhalation) to that when the lungs are filled with air. However, people with large chests breathe no more effectively than those people with average-sized chests who use their breathing organs efficiently to spread oxygen throughout their bodies.

Chest Breathing: the body undertakes this natural method only during strenuous exertion. It might be termed a form of *forced breathing.* It is an emergency measure. Unfortunately, most people rob themselves of oxygen when they breathe, because they use only a minimum of the top portion of their lungs.

Diaphragmatic Breathing: this is the natural method designed for the body. When you inhale, the diaphragm expands. It not only expands the chest cavity and draws air into the lungs, but it also expands the abdominal cavity. It does more than just drawing in air, it stretches and massages the abdominal muscles and organs. When you exhale the diaphragm relaxes. It expels air from the lungs, exercises the rib muscles and massages the heart. Because this tones and tightens the abdominal muscles, you get healthier with each super power breath!

Wake up and say, "Today I am going to be happier, healthier and wiser in my daily living. I am the captain of my life and am going to steer it for 100% healthy lifestyle living!" Fact: Happy people look younger, have fewer health problems and live longer! – Patricia Bragg, ND, PhD, Pioneer Health Crusader

Harmonious, Rhythmic Breathing massages the heart, liver and pancreas & helps improve functions of spleen, stomach, small intestine & abdomen. Your nerves will be calm, your voice will relax & your face will shine with a soft, healthy glow.

Internal Massage by Diaphragmatic Action

The diaphragm's effect on the muscles and organs of the abdomen is highly beneficial. To combat the pull of gravity and hold the abdominal organs in place, our abdominal muscles need all the exercise we can find time to give them. Correct, natural diaphragmatic breathing – along with daily exercise and practicing good posture (pages 169-176) – helps to accomplish many health miracles.

Your diaphragmatic natural action also provides an important massage for the heart, chest and stomach areas, and the liver, intestines, kidneys, gallbladder, spleen and pancreas. This stimulates blood circulation and helps these organs to perform the functions which are essential to maintaining your life and your health for a long life!

The dual action of the diaphragm, which affects the upper thoracic organs (heart and lungs) and the lower abdominal organs, is a vital factor in good blood circulation. This is especially true as blood returns through the veins to the heart. The forceful pumping thrust of the heart muscles sends blood coursing through the arteries. This force is almost spent by the time the bloodstream has dispensed oxygen, nutrients and collected wastes, and is ready to return to the heart through the veins. The return trip is dependent upon the contraction of the muscles and muscular walls of the viscera – the internal organs contained within the abdominal and thoracic cavities. The rhythmic massage of the abdominal organs by the respiratory muscles plays a pivotal role in this vital return of blood to the heart.

Diaphragmatic breathing stimulates the *peristalsis,* the wavelike-squeezing motion of the intestines which promotes digestion and the elimination of solid and semi-solid fecal wastes. Making a change from chest breathing to diaphragmatic breathing has helped thousands in correcting heartburn, indigestion, gas, chronic constipation, and liver problems, etc.

Deep Healthy Breathing: *is about 10-12 breaths per minute, from the diaphragm (rather than the chest), through the nose (rather than mouth) and is quiet and light. Deep breathing techniques increase oxygenation!* – NaturalNews.com

Bragg Super Power Breathing Calms the Nervous System

The *solar plexus* is the *powerhouse* of the body. It's a network of nerves and ganglia (independent groups of nerve cells) which controls every important vital organ in the abdominal cavity and is located in the very center of the diaphragm. The more stimulation you give your diaphragm, the more circulation your solar plexus (often called the gut) receives. This increases the amount of nerve energy that is then available to your vital organs. The extremely important pneumogastric nerve (*pneuma* – lungs; *gastro* – stomach) passes through the diaphragm and also benefits from this diaphragmatic action.

Diaphragmatic breathing has a tranquilizing rhythm, stimulates your circulation and helps rejuvenate the body. B-complex vitamins also have a calming effect on the entire nervous system. Diaphragmatic breathing breaks up the paralyzing nerve tension so often observed in people with supersensitive or jangled nerves. For more details about the beneficial effects of deep breathing on the nerves, do read our book *Build Powerful Nerve Force*. (See pages 237-239 for more information on Bragg Books.)

Yoga teaches that deep, rhythmic breathing attunes one to the *rhythm of the universe* – in other words, one lives in rhythmic harmony with Mother Nature. *Prana*, the Sanskrit word for *breath*, also means *absolute energy* or *vital cosmic energy*. According to the teachings of yoga, when we breathe correctly we store this energy in the solar plexus.

The Ayurvedic Health and Fitness Lifestyle

An ancient healing system developed in India many thousands of years ago, Ayurveda (means science of life) and is reemerging with their therapies for health and fitness, yoga, herbs, etc. In the ancient teachings of Ayurveda, a person's mind-body type is determined, then specific diet, exercise and lifestyle routines are prescribed that are best for them, according to their mind and body type.

You are where you are because you want to be there. If you want to be somewhere else, you'll need to change. – Mark Victor Hansen, Co-Producer, "Chicken Soup" Series

I strive to be pure and good in all things – in body, mind and soul. – Paul C. Bragg

Ancient Yoga Breathing Promotes Health

Essential to Ayurveda is the daily practice of yoga stretching and the importance of breathing correctly. Yoga breathing helps the mind and body become one. Learning to breathe correctly helps you remain calm in your daily living, during exercise and in stressful times.

Yoga breathing is nose breathing. For centuries, this has been known to slow the heart, lower blood pressure and relieve stress. Because it is a more efficient way to get oxygen into your body, it will enhance athletic performance. To practice it, start by doing some yoga stretches. Then walk with gradually increasing speed – breathing only through your nose – until you are jogging. When you can no longer nose-breathe easily, slow down until you can again breathe comfortably through your nose. Do this back and forth several times – jogging, walking, etc., always breathing through your nose. Finish with enjoyable yoga stretches. Practiced regularly, this calms you and gives you a greater oxygen capacity intake and increased energy, health and vitality. See website: *www.HealthAndYoga.com.*

The Benefits of Full Yoga Breathing

- Releases acute & chronic muscular tensions in the body, especially around the heart & digestive organs.
- Increases lung capacity – this helps asthma & emphysema sufferers overcome their fear of having shortness of breath attacks.
- Encourages proper nervous stimulus to the cardio-vascular system.
- Dramatically reduces emotional & nervous anxiety.
- Improves detox by increased carbon dioxide and oxygen exchange.
- Helps auto immune system by increased energy to endocrine system that regulates metabolism, tissue function, internal temperature, water balance, ions and moods.
- Calms the mind & integrates the mental & physical balance.
- Contributes to both vitality, energy, & relaxation.

  With such powerful all-round benefits, do you really need to be "motivated" to get going? Go ahead, and take charge of your life like never before. – Courtesy: www.HealthAndYoga.com

THE BREATH BUILDER®: An exercise tool for anyone who recognizes the value of deep breathing. Used regularly, the Breath Builder exerciser will increase the amount of air you inhale and exhale. It can benefit anyone . . . but especially helpful for persons suffering from emphysema or any other breathing problems. The Breath Builder will bring new life to the body, new energy to the spirit and new gusto to living! Available on website: www.stretching.com

No One Can Breathe for You

You can build a new figure, a new You – inside and out – vibrant, healthy and tingling with the joy of life. Remember, You and You Alone have this great power to breathe deeply – You are Your Captain, it's all up to You!

This self-power to breathe deeply has no value unless it is used every day. You can build better blood circulation by daily doing The Bragg Super Power Breathing exercises and living The Bragg Healthy Lifestyle. You will soon become oxygen recharged and not feel fatigued at the least physical effort. Prove this to yourself – start today!

Breathing exercises bring sparkle to your eyes, a glow to your flesh and add vim and vigor to your step. You will be more mentally alert. Your reflexes will function better. You will feel more fit with a sense of well-being that is a far greater treasure than any material possession!

Oxygen is the most valuable of all nature's elements and you can have all you can breathe for free. You have only to learn how to fully utilize it with Bragg Super Power Breathing. By practicing long, slow breathing and taking longer, deeper breaths per minute you will enjoy greater health, more endurance, vitality, energy and a youthful life!

Breathing deeply gives you more energy, go-power and sparkles up your life!
– Paul C. Bragg, N.D., Ph.D., Health Crusader & Lifestyle Educator

Chapter 8

Super Power Breathing –
Your Way to Health & Happiness

Your lungs can hold at least 6 pints of air. If you keep your lungs filled to capacity you will feel better, have more energy, suffer less fatigue, sleep better, wake up refreshed and be a healthier, happier person. With practice you can easily learn to control your breathing, taking only 6 to 8 long, full breaths per minute for a healthier and more energized productive life. Prove it – start now!

Super Oxygen Breathing for Super Living

When your body is fed with Live Foods and Super Oxygen, the joy of living will thrill you. Every day you bounce out of bed with a glad to be alive feeling, knowing there is meaning in life. You'll have fewer depressing thoughts, feelings, envy, jealousies, blue Mondays, hatreds, anger, frustrations, fears, worries or morbid feelings!

With the stimulation of Super Oxygen, you are eager to meet life's problems. You meet them face to face and find solutions. You enjoy the effort of facing life's realities. You fully use the intelligence and commonsense God gave you. Those people who know how to breathe deeply do not run away from life, but face it with courage and determination. The weakling, inevitably a shallow breather, takes the escape offered by alcohol, drugs and self-pity that leads to illness.

Look at your life. Has it become overly complex? Have you found yourself burdened by too many possessions or responsibilities? Take a slow, deep breath and ask: "What steps can I take to reduce clutter so I may live life simply and joyously?"
– Douglas Bloch, M.A., author, teacher & counselor • HealingFromDepression.com

Some of life's greatest pleasures happen when we slow down, and enjoy the little things that brighten life. – Mac Anderson

We are a product of our thoughts – and so is our health! While doctors and medicine have their place, self-healing is the most powerful medicine of all. Accepting the present and placing trust in a higher power frees your energy to focus on improving your life! See problems as challenges of growth, not as a punishment or judgement! Focus on happiness, forgiveness, hope and peace of mind, as well as physical change to ease any problems and situations.

Deep Breathing and Walk Worries Away!

You can truly *walk your worries away!* As the blood (*your river of life*) courses through your arteries and veins, cleansing and nourishing your entire body, you become filled with a sense of well-being. This cleanses your mind of its troubles and nourishes it with positive, healthy, happy thoughts.

Enjoy your walk with a free spirit and a light heart. Start at your own pace to fit the movement – fast, medium or slow. Watch with interest the things and people you pass, or let your walking be an accompaniment to your ideas and thoughts. As you breathe and walk rhythmically, awareness of your body will diminish. You will become more at peace and happier and in tune with Mother Earth and God.

As we stride along on our brisk walks we say, "Health, Strength, Youth, Vitality, Peace, Love, Joy, Eternity!" With walking you discover the beauty of God and Mother Nature as it awakens, softens and enriches your soul and life!

Deep Breathing Key to Healthy, Happy Life!

Health and happiness may reside in your brain, and more specifically with the power of your breath. You may be surprised to learn that recent advances and studies in "mind-body medicine" offer a deeper understanding of how something as simple as your breath could be the answer to your health, happiness and longevity!

Most of us do shallow, anxious, quick breathing . . . not connecting our breath deep into the diaphragm. Deep breathing has now been shown in many studies to have a significant benefit on calming and soothing both mind and body. When you connect and focus on your breath by taking deep and slow inhalations and exhalations, your nervous system and brain waves begin to come into balance.

Many ancient healing traditions, such as Yoga, meditation and Tai Chi, have recognized that one of the simplest and most effective tools we have to create more happiness in our life is to do deep breathing exercises. Recent medical studies suggest that deep, conscious, breathing might have the same effects as anti-depressant medication! Info from web: *DrJayKumar.com*

50

Man's precious breath is the gift of life from God.
With the care and nurturing of this life gift, all health and wisdom is ours.

Can Deep Breathing Influence Your Happiness?

Deep breathing engages the diaphragm, the muscle which divides your chest from abdomen. On an inhale, the diaphragm moves down to allow the lungs to expand with oxygen. On the exhale, the diaphragm presses up against the lungs to dispel carbon dioxide.

Most of us slip into the habit of breathing with the upper half of our lungs. Our intercostal muscles get a workout, but our belly barely moves. Inside the chest, this means the lower lobes of our lungs don't get a full helping of fresh oxygen. According to Harvard Medical School, many small blood vessels instrumental in carrying oxygen to cells reside in the lowest portion of the lungs. When these areas are deprived of air, you can feel short of breath and anxious – which is the opposite of feeling happy.

Deep breathing stimulates the parasympathetic nervous system, which guides the body from stress to relaxation. When we're relaxed, our heart rate and blood pressure lowers, and our digestion and health improves.

By training yourself to breathe slowly and deeply in your everyday life, you're priming your body to relax. You're turning off the "fight-or-flight" response that occurs when you're stressed, and giving yourself more opportunities to slow down, think clearly, be thankful, and happy and healthy. It all begins one breath at a time!

Breathing is the greatest pleasure in life – it gives life! – Papini, 1881-1956

There is a positive side and a negative side and at every moment you can decide. – Sister Corita

During your weekly 24 hour fast try to avoid criticizing anyone or anything! Fill yourself only with loving, positive thoughts, not only on your fasting and cleansing days, but everyday! Before you speak put your words to this test! "Is it good? Is it kind? Is it necessary? If not, don't speak!" – Patricia Bragg, ND, PhD.

Taking deep breaths gets more oxygen into your lungs and helps improve drainage of your lymphatic system, which removes toxins from your body. Deep Breathing helps in stress relief. Slow, rhythmic, deep breathing acts as a mini meditation. Shift to slower breathing in times of tension – inhale for four counts and exhale for eight – it helps to de-stress and energize you at the same time!
– Dr. Oz • www.DrOz.com

The health of the people is really the foundation upon which all their happiness and all their powers as a state depend. – Benjamin Disraeli, Britain Prime Minister

Breathing Right Contributes to Happiness!

Breathing is your body's most essential requirement for life. Without oxygen, you would only live a few minutes at most. But your breath is more than just simple movements of oxygen in and out of your lungs. It is necessary for your body functions. The air you breathe has its own energy fields or life force. This life force is in all living things on Earth. Without it, we would not be alive at all. It's this very life force, which is a combination of electric and magnetic energies and more that is keeping our heart, lungs, kidneys, liver and all other organs pumping and functioning through electrical signals received from the brain. – *NaturalNews.com*

A proper breathing pattern will allow you to wake up rested, keep your energy levels balanced throughout the day, decrease your waistline by improving digestion, and slow down your cellular metabolism so that you can live a long, happy life. Because your breath mirrors your mental state, you can guide your breath to become calm and slow. Calming your breath also calms the thoughts in your mind. and thereby making your mind even quieter.

Breathing slowly and deeply can lead you into more peaceful spaces within your mind, heart and soul.

Once you develop deep breathing by practicing it every day, twice a day, it will be a very useful tool that you will always have with you. Use it whenever anything upsetting happens – before you react. Use it whenever you are aware of internal tension. Use it to help you fall asleep. Use it to deal with food cravings. Great for mild to moderate anxiety, this exercise cannot be recommended too highly. Everyone can benefit from it.

If you are honest with yourself, you will quickly discover that most of the things you truly love to do in your leisure time are not only simple, but also free and surprisingly healthy. So, instead of rushing out to see the latest film or show, why not watch the sunset? Take a walk in nature alone or with a loved one! Read the Bible, a favorite book or listen to your favorite music! Relax and enjoy!

Breathing deeply, fully and completely energizes the body, calms the nerves, fills you with peace and helps keep you youthful. – Paul C. Bragg, ND, PhD.

Miracles can happen every day through guidance and prayer!
– Patricia Bragg, ND, PhD., Pioneer Health Crusader

Chapter 9

Powerful Benefits of Bragg Super Power Breathing

A Strong Mind in A Strong Healthy Body

Ancient Greek civilization, which produced some of the greatest minds the world has known, lived by the motto: *A strong mind in a strong body*. The Ancient Greeks were noted for their amazing powers of endurance, robust health and youthful longevity! All of these were the results of their systems of natural eating, deep breathing and strenuous exercise, which produced physiques that have served as the models of classical art ever since.

The classic Greeks followed 4 main health principles:

1. Full, deep, super power breathing.
2. Eating two meals of natural, healthy foods per day.
3. Exercise regime for complete body development.
4. They honored supreme health, body, mind and soul.

We can do the same and achieve the same results they did. We can become more vital and totally fit – enjoying every minute of being alive! The time to start is NOW – whatever your calendar years. Whether you are a teenager or a great-grandparent or somewhere in between, it is never too early or too late to start on your Supreme Road to Super Health!

GLOOM

SUNSHINE

ROAD TO ILLNESS   ROAD TO HEALTH

DEAD END

NEGATIVE ⇦ **OR** ⇨ **POSITIVE**
The choice of which road to take is up to you.

You alone decide whether to reach a dead end or live a healthy lifestyle for a long, healthy, happy, active life. – Paul C. Bragg

Super Power Breathing Promotes Healthy Body

The most important of all physical acts is correct breathing. The rhythm and depth of your breath directly affects the state of your mind and the health of your body. You can not be 100% healthy if you don't breathe deeply. Taking deeper breaths will bring in more oxygen into your body and improve your energy levels! Deep breathing is not only important for living longer but also to have a good mood and keep performing at your best.

Here's benefits of deep breathing and why you should make it a part of your daily living.

✳ *Deep Breathing Detoxifies and Releases Toxins.* The body is designed to release 70% of its toxins through breathing. If you are not breathing effectively, you are not ridding your body of toxins. Then the other systems of your body must work overtime which could eventually lead to illness.

✳ *All Internal Organs are Massaged.* The movements of the diaphragm during deep breathing exercise massages the stomach, small intestine, liver and the pancreas.

✳ *Respiratory System Works Better.* Difficulties such as asthma, bronchitis and other respiratory systems and even chest pain can subside (see info on pages 83-94).

✳ *Digestive System Does Its Job.* Digestive ills (poor digestion, bloating, constipation) are helped by the internal massage of correct diaphragmatic action. When a Super Power Breath is taken, digestive tract gets healthy exercise. Deep optimal breathing is the great body health normalizer. Oxygen, the invisible staff of life, is food for the body and helps with assimilation of foods. Oxygen burns calories and helps promote normal, healthy weight. The digestive organs receive more oxygen, and hence operate more efficiently.

"To stop heartburn, gerds, indigestion and improve digestion, sip ¹/₂ tsp Bragg's Organic Apple Cider Vinegar before meals." – Dr. Gabriel Cousens, MD, Author of "Conscious Eating"

Stop Chewing Gum Habit– It Causes Stomach and Digestive Problems: *Please never chew gum – it fools the body into thinking food is coming. Chewing starts digestive juices flowing. These powerful juices can cause trouble with your empty stomach's lining, resulting in stomach ulcer problems, heartburn, bloating, gas, etc.*

�֍ *Lymph System Works Better.* Increases circulation of lymphatic fluid which speeds recovery after illnesses.

�֍ *Circulation System Moves!* Many people suffer from poor circulation in various parts of the body. Because they don't get sufficient oxygen to produce a steady blood circulation into their extremities, they have cold hands, feet, noses and ears. The more oxygen you get into your body, it's better for your circulation, heart, and your hands and feet will be warmer! When more oxygen gets into your bloodstream, you will feel super energized and have greater super vitality to better enjoy a longer, healthier, happier life! See web: *breathing.com*

✷ *Immune System has More Energy.* Deep Breathing creates more energy for the body to heal and detoxify. Helps tissues to regenerate and heal. Enriches your blood cells to metabolize nutrients and vitamins. Super Power Breathing is now a part of all cures. Today, in the modern hospital, pure oxygen heals when every other method of healing has failed. Even broken bones heal more quickly when the blood is purified by doing daily Super Power Breathing Exercises. Oxygen – the great invisible food for life, stimulant and purifier – builds our health resistance to infections and strengthens our weak points. It's God's most vital aid in helping the body to heal itself and to stay healthy!

✷ *Cleansing Systems Works Better.* Excess fluids are eliminated through deep breathing. The stress on organs is lessened, allowing the body to cleanse naturally.

✷ *Blood Quality Improves.* When you regularly breathe oxygen correctly, you are adding millions of health-giving, oxygen-carrying red blood cells to your bloodstream, your miracle river of life. Deep Breathing removes all the carbon-dioxide and increases oxygen in the blood.

✷ *Nervous System Improves.* Brain, spinal cord and nerves receive increased oxygen. This improves the health of the whole body, since the nervous system communicates to all parts of the body. Many nervous diseases are due to oxygen starvation. Deep, diaphragmatic breathing tranquilizes jangled nerves, stimulates brain with clear thinking and more alertness to help solve any life problems and make wise decisions (see more page 58).

✳ *Lungs are Strengthened.* When you fill your lungs with more miracle-working oxygen, you cleanse your body of toxic poisons that could do your body great health damage. As you breathe deeply the lungs become healthier and more powerful. Good insurance against respiratory problems.

✳ *Heart Grows Stronger.* Slow, deep breaths soothe and recharge the heart. Conversely, rapid, shallow breathing exhausts it through overwork and lack of sufficient oxygen for the blood. Since the heart doesn't have to work as hard to deliver oxygen to the tissues, the heart can rest a little.

✳ *Muscles Get a Workout.* When you breathe easier you move easier! Deep breathing increases flexibility and strengthens joints. Supplies oxygen to brain and all cells in your body which increases the muscles in your body.

✳ *Emotionally You Feel Better.* People who deeply inhale larger amounts of oxygen are happier people. Super Power Breathing cleanses your body of psychological and physical poisons and gives you more joyful daily living and also more emotional well-being (see pages 50-52).

✳ *Reduces Feelings of Stress.* Deep breathing relaxes the body and releases endorphins – natural pain-killers that create natural highs – and makes it easier to sleep. Deep breathing will help clear uneasy feelings out of your body.

✳ *You Become Mentally Present.* Mental observation and concentration is improved. There is greater productivity, insight and learning and better decision making.

✳ *Physical Appearance Improves.* People who get ample oxygen sleep better and have better muscle tone. Skin is healthier, firmer and more alive! Oxygen is Mother Nature's great miracle beautifier. It gives the skin a radiant glow and the hair a lustrous sheen.

You will have less wrinkles from improved circulation. Breathing helps create beautiful skin at any age! Good breathing techniques will also encourage good posture, which in turn helps you to look and feel younger (see posture exercise page 173). If you are overweight, the extra oxygen helps burn up excess fat more efficiently.

There are only two ways to live your life. One way is as though nothing is a miracle. The other way is as everything is a miracle! – Albert Einstein

Deep breathing increases the flow of blood and oxygen to heart, brain & eyes.

* *Increases Your Spirituality.* Deep Breathing deepens your meditation and increases your intuition when you're relaxed. Helps connect you to your inner soul which helps with "self-love" and greater compassion for others.

* *Promotes Super Energy!* You will no longer crave artificial stimulants (caffeine, alcohol, tobacco) when sufficient oxygen is taken into your system. Oxygen is the wise stimulant that has no harmful after-effects.

Deep, Full Breathing Helps Relieve Pain

Civilized human beings with their unhealthy, self-destructive eating and living habits tend to accumulate latent poisons in their bodies. This means that the body stockpiles toxic poisons in different areas when they could not be disposed of through the body's regular avenues of elimination. These poisons are stored in veins, arteries, joints, organs, tissues, skin, etc. When they accumulate and press on nerves and tissues, there is pain. You may think this pain is new, but it's usually a *flare-up* of the old stored-up body toxins (except in cases of injury).

Heed Body's Warning Pains – Eliminate Cause

Don't take pills to ease warning pains – find cause and eliminate it! Live The Bragg Healthy Lifestyle! Use oxygen to help flush poisons out of your body! There's absolutely no better way of flushing toxic poisons out of the body than by the powerful action of oxygen. Ample power breathing, 8 glasses of pure distilled water daily (3 of them add Bragg Apple Cider Vinegar, page 149), and fasting, are the greatest natural purifiers on earth! For instance, you may have a pain in your right foot which is quite common, since the force of gravity will often cause toxins to settle in the legs and feet. Painful gout is perfect example of this tendency.

Man is the sole and absolute master of his own fate forever. What he has sown in times of ignorance, he must inevitably reap; when he attains enlightenment, it is for him to sow what he chooses and reap accordingly.
– Sir Walter Scott, Scottish Poet

The three greatest letters in the English alphabet are N-O-W.
There is no time like the present. Begin Now! – Sir Walter Scott, Scottish Poet

---

Oxygen plays vital role, not only in our breathing process but in every metabolic process in the body. Nutrient compounds inside our cells are oxidized by enzymes and this process is our main source of energy. – NaturalNews.com

Now let's get the toxins out of that right foot! Exercise as follows: lie flat on back, take a long, deep breath and hold it. While holding your breath, raise left leg, bend at knee, and with both hands pull and press your leg against your chest as you exert the full downward force of your diaphragm at the same time. You will feel oxygenated blood flowing unrestricted down into your right foot. Now slowly exhale. (Also it's wise never sit with legs crossed.)

This same technique may be applied to any part of the body. For example, for a headache, take a full breath (exhaling and inhaling as in Exercise 1, page 72). Holding the breath, relax your shoulders and bend your head downward below your heart. This allows a free flow of oxygenated blood to the cavities of the head and brain. Headaches are also helped by fasting and the herb Feverfew.

Aches and pains from fatigue are nearly always due to stagnant venous blood filled with toxic carbon dioxide and congestion in various parts of the body. Swollen ankles, can occur due to an unhealthy diet, salt, etc. and build-up of venous blood and water bloating. Exercise and Super Power Breathing will help to activate circulation and return blood to the heart. From the heart it will be pumped to the lungs, where the carbon dioxide will be expelled and exchanged for body purifying oxygen.

B-Complex, Magnesium and Deep Breathing Improves Brain Function and Soothes Nerve

When an emotional upset occurs, which inevitably befalls each of us, go off by yourself and take long, slow, relaxed breaths. Soon you'll find your nerves quieting down and more logical thinking will replace emotionalism. You will become master of the situation and better able to calmly resolve your problem. (Magnesium, B12, B-Complex or their injections help breathing, calm nerves and improve brain function. St. John's Wort also helps.) Read our book *Build Powerful Nerve Force* (pages 237-239) for info on improving nerve health.

Better an ounce of prevention, than a pound of cure!
Start now to breathe deeply and live fully!

Now I see the secret of making the best persons, it is to grow in the open air, live simple and eat natural foods and sleep with Mother Earth. – Walt Whitman

Deep Breathing Helps Respiratory Ailments

Letters and case stories give testimony to the blessed relief that Bragg Super Power Breathing has brought to thousands suffering from breathing problems such as sinusitis, bronchitis, asthma and emphysema. These suffocating diseases, characterized by chronic mucus inflammation and obstruction of the air passages, have become more prevalent today as our air becomes more polluted. (Take precaution, use air purifiers and humidifiers for home, office and your car, see page 119.) In fact, colds, flu and chronic sinus inflammation are the most common illnesses seen by doctors today (backaches are second).

Breathing Exercises Stimulate Pituitary Gland

Stimulation of the body's master gland, the pituitary, is one of the greatest benefits of Bragg Super Power Breathing Exercises. *The pituitary gland is located at the base of the brain and is the master miracle of every human act and unconscious function occurring within the heart and abdominal cavity.* It determines a person's height, length of their bones, muscle and pulse strength, mental activity and even lifespan.

The pituitary is the master gland of life and controls the functions of all other body glands. The more oxygenated blood you give the pituitary gland, the greater output of all valuable body hormones. The better the glands function, the more the entire body will rejuvenate itself to stay healthier and more youthful!

This is why the following exercises are called Super Power Breathing Exercises. Although each one is directed toward a specific part of the body, all employ the same basic, super oxygen principle. They all also stimulate the master pituitary gland and brain area with super oxygen.

Minimizing your exposure to environmental toxins (ex. using air and water purifiers, eating organic foods, etc.) while restoring oxygen balance in the body is a commonsense plan for cellular rejuvenation and disease prevention. These are simple ways to improve oxygenation in your body! – NaturalNews.com

---

Improper breathing is common cause of ill health. Changing & improving your breathing patterns can affect you emotionally & physically. – www.DrWeil.com

59

Mother Nature Loves You To Enjoy Her Beauty

Let me look upward
into the branches
Of the towering oak
And know that it grew
slowly and well.

Give me, amidst
the confusion
of my day
The calmness of
the everlasting hills.

Let me pause
to look at a flower,
to smell a rose —
God's autograph,
to chat with a friend,
to read a few lines
from a good book.

Break the tensions
of my nerves
With the soothing music
of singing streams
and gentle rains
That live in
my memory.

Follow steps of the godly,
and stay on the right path
to enjoy life to the fullest.
— Proverbs 2:20-21

60

Open your eyes to behold wondrous things out of Thy law. – Psalm 119:18

Chapter 10

Preparing for Bragg Super Power Breathing

What is Bragg Super Power Breathing?

Bragg Super Power Breathing is based upon simple, natural laws. The more oxygen you get into the body, the more carbon dioxide poison you will eliminate from the body. When oxygen replaces carbon dioxide, there will be greater purification of the blood, cells and organs of the body for improved better health and a longer life!

Thousands upon thousands of lives have been saved with oxygen therapy! It is a well established scientific fact that, when all known conventional methods of healing fail, oxygen thereby is used to save lives. So, if pure oxygen can save the lives of humans who are on the brink of death, is it not logical that inhaling more oxygen deeply can prolong our lives? Or that it will free us from toxins that bring pain and distress to our physical bodies and give us a greater enjoyment of life?

Oxygen is the only stimulant upon which you can safely rely as a depression chaser and body builder. Bragg Super Power Breathing's main purpose is to get more life-giving oxygen into all parts of your body for health.

Bragg Super Power Breathing Exercises should not be confused with physical exercises. While this kind of breathing does produce more energy and physical and nerve strength, it has nothing to do with mere muscular development. However, it is almost impossible to have ample oxygen freely circulating in the body without beneficial effects occurring throughout. Extra benefits will be healthier muscle tone, more firmness of the skin and improved posture. Oxygen is a miracle normalizer!

The basic principle of Bragg Super Power Breathing is to fill the lungs to capacity with oxygen, then hold breath in, leaning forward, drop your head below your heart. This uses the force of gravity to infuse the head's cavities with oxygenated blood, which energizes brain, helps maintain and create new brain cells (see Salk Institute page 16).

Overcoming the Effects of Bad Breathing

The Bragg Breathing Exercises and Healthy Lifestyle work to tone and regulate your entire body to make it healthier. Most humans are victims of two bad habits: shallow breathing and incorrect posture and must be overcome! Muscles must be strengthened, especially the diaphragm and the abdominal muscles. Unused lung air sacs must be opened and revitalized fully with oxygen.

Perhaps you have already experienced a *stitch in the side* when you have had to run to catch a bus or plane, or while doing some unaccustomed exercise. Actually this can be a good sign, if you will profit by it. It is good to exercise to the point of getting that *stitch*. What it really means is that you have discovered a large area of unused lung cells, which have remained closed most of your life, since childhood. Now your lungs are opening to receive the fresh air you are pumping in through your efforts to breathe more deeply. The diaphragms of older people can become semi-paralyzed from non-use, but with exercise and Bragg Deep Super Power Breathing that can change!

As lung cells suffer disuse they begin to stick together and collapse in upon themselves. The sharp pain is due to the air forcing these cells apart. Continue to breathe deeply, even after you have caught the bus, plane or stopped your exercise, run, etc. The distress soon passes and your unused lung cells will soon become reactivated! You will then have made an important step forward in Bragg Super Power Breathing and achieving greater super vitality and health.

If you experience that *stitch* during the preparatory exercises which we are going to outline, you will now understand what it is caused by and not be alarmed. Just keep doing your deep breathing for more super energy!

Breathing is the greatest pleasure in life – it gives life! – Papini, 1881-1956

TEST See if you are a chest breather or abdomen breather: Place right hand on chest and left hand on abdomen. As you breathe, see which hand rises more. If right hand rises more, you are a chest breather. If left hand rises more, you are an abdomen breather. – See web: www.LiveStrong.com.

Remember: "It is NEVER too late to be what you might have been!"

Breathe Through the Mouth and the Nose

To breathe most effectively one should use both the mouth and nose to breathe. Our Creator has equipped our noses with miracle hair filters to strain out dust and pollens. It also has temperature regulating chambers (sinuses) to warm or cool the air before it enters the lungs, as well as moist mucus which traps particles missed by the hairs and expels them through the nose or mouth. The human body is also equipped with a larger, secondary air entrance, the mouth for use when a greater amount of oxygen is needed: during strenuous sports and exercise such as swimming, running, or bicycling.

Since the purpose of Bragg Super Power Breathing is to fill the lungs with as much oxygen as possible, we use both the nose and mouth to breathe in and out. Do this breathing exercise often – fill your lungs by breathing deeply in through the nose; pucker lips into a small opening; now exhale slowly and strongly with a hissing sound.

Fresh Air and Warmth are Necessary

Sleep in a well-ventilated (airy) room on a firm mattress. Use natural cotton percale or flannel sheets, also these and silk are preferred for bedtime wear, or wear nothing. Don't use electric blankets or heating pads, because they can disturb body's natural currents, even be harmful to health, state scientists. If you must, only use to pre-warm, then unplug! Safer to fill empty Bragg Vinegar bottle with hot water.

Be sure there's ample fresh air circulating in your room. If not, do these exercises before an open window. We want you to get full benefit of these stimulating breathing exercises and to enjoy every minute of them. If it's too cool when you get out of bed, put on something that is loose and warm. We often wear cozy sweatshirts and sweatpants.

As you start doing your exercises you will soon feel a wonderful glow of circulation coming over your entire body as you become warmer. When you feel warm enough, peel off your sweat clothes and get right down to your bare skin. Remember that you also breathe through your skin! It's an important organ of respiration – your skin and billions of pores are often called your *third lung.*

Air Baths are Health Builders

Give yourself an external as well as an internal air bath. Let your approximately 2 billion pores breathe in the breath of life, too. The pores of your body will welcome the contact with fresh air. They are wrapped up in clothes all day and probably at night also, unless you sleep in the nude. Daily air baths (babies love them too) do wonders for the skin. No creams can give you *"skin you love to touch"* like fresh air can! A daily private (nude) air bath also greatly enhances your skin's primary function as the main thermostatic regulator (control) of your body's temperature. This practice helps condition the skin to adjust to hot and cold weather more easily. It's a faithful thermostat when you treat it well. But if you keep your body heavily clothed and overheated all the time, your skin becomes like a hothouse plant, unable to withstand drastic temperature changes. When you allow your entire body to breathe freely in the nude, your body's thermostat learns to readjust itself so that it works perfectly for you in hot and cold weather! (Also, try this powerful combination 2-3 times weekly: air bath and light skin brushing – page 211.)

Enjoy Early Morning Breathing Exercises

Upon awakening in the morning it's ideal to first do some slow body stretching exercises. Then super-charge your day with a peak supply of oxygen energy by doing 10-15 minutes of Super Power Breathing Exercises. After your exercises enjoy a glass of our delicious Bragg Apple Cider Vinegar Drink (1-2 tsps ACV mixed with 1-2 tsps raw honey (optional) in a glass of distilled water, recipe on page 149). For more info read these 2 books: *Apple Cider Vinegar –Miracle Health System* and *Water – The Shocking Truth That Can Save Your Life!* (Bragg book list pages 237-239.)

The early morning hours are especially important for doing these breathing exercises, especially if a city dweller, because air is less polluted then. These exercises will super start your day with super energy that will carry you through whatever challenges may arise. You will become more confident, stronger and healthier.

Think of this health-building period with pleasant anticipation. It's a time to build your vitality, energy, strength and all the good things that come to a healthy body. Go into it with dedicated self-responsibility and enthusiasm. Your faithful efforts will bring super results!

Practice Bragg Posture Exercises Every Day

Correct posture (see page 171) allows chest to expand so the lungs can be filled with air. The lungs inflate with air like millions of tiny balloons. Suction is created below by the action of the diaphragm and above by the auxiliary muscles of the chest and abdomen. This suction fills your lungs with air. The lungs themselves are passive and cannot breathe independently. The lungs wait patiently to be refilled with air. So now make it a habit to breathe deeply to help keep your lungs and body healthy.

Remember, the lungs are attached to the rib cage walls by pleural membranes. If the sternum, or breastbone, is carried high and the bony rib cage expanded, the lungs are held up with good posture so they can be easily filled with air. The uplifted diaphragm, in turn, tends to draw into position any sagging or prolapsed stomach organs.

As with deep breathing, most young children exhibit good posture naturally, only to lose both as they mature! To make matters worse, most occupations today (from assembly line to desk jobs) have a tendency to pull us down from an erect, good posture position. The result is that many people carry themselves like a collapsed accordion, shoulders sagging, chest deflated, which puts their heart, organs and breathing apparatus in a tight viselike grip!

1 See posture exercise (page 173) to help counteract this unhealthy and energy-sapping poor posture. Now stand with feet 10" apart and stretch hands high overhead, at same time rising high on toes. See how high you can lift up your chest while drawing in abdominal muscles. Stretch up and up, as if trying to touch the ceiling. *Now drop arms. Relax and repeat this exercise 10 times.* Do not try to do any special breathing. Just breathe naturally, or what is natural for you at the time.

He who can't find time for exercise will have time for illness. – Lord Derby

This stretching exercise is designed to strengthen the muscles which control the erect posture of the body. Stretching is one of the greatest tools for building health. It is the universal exercise of the animal kingdom. Wild animals are beautiful examples of instinctual natural living. Also, your pets (cats, dogs, birds, etc.) all wisely stretch daily. *When you sit awhile, stand up and do some stretching exercises!*

Stomach Muscles Need These Exercises

Most people allow their stomach muscles to be lazy, flabby and unhealthy. Carrying excess belly fat around waistline can impair lung function (*reuters.com*). Abdominal obesity is defined as having a waistline of greater than 35 inches for women and 40 inches for men. The French researchers think belly fat may impair the way the diaphragm and chest function. A good time to strengthen, tone and control these natural girdle muscles is to practice these two exercises every morning before getting out of bed. Remember your waistline is your lifeline!

2 Lying on your back – fix your eyes and attention on your stomach. Now start moving your stomach muscles upwards, then force them downwards. Wiggle your insides, in one direction, then another, then from side to side, letting your hands help at first. When you discover you can control your stomach muscles in one movement, then practice the other movements. Do daily for results!

Thinking about and using these stomach muscles is just the beginning. The goal of these exercises is the ability to control the abdominal muscles in the same way you do those of the legs and arms. Your stomach muscles must do your bidding if you want to develop a useful diaphragm. After you have obtained some control over your stomach muscles while lying on your back in bed, *begin doing the same movements while standing upright.* You can accomplish much more with your muscles in this upright position.

3 Standing upright, with hands hanging relaxed at sides, draw in and up the stomach muscles until it looks like a deep valley, as though everything inside was moving

Your waistline is your healthline, dateline, youthline and lifeline! – Patricia Bragg

up in the chest cavity. Then push your muscles out until you see your protruding belly. Now suck the muscles in, then push out. Now wiggle them up and down, and last pull in, tighten, firm and stretch up your midsection and spine. Repeat several times. This is called Nauli Kriya.

When you acquire this control over the abdomen and surrounding muscles, you will discover many benefits. Abdominal exercises strengthen the body and result in a straight, aligned spine. With a strong mid-section, the body can stand tall. Another reward is it helps you establish a more normal bowel rhythm. Usually soon after arising and within an hour after each meal there should be a bowel movement. (See simple exercise bottom page 74.)

Diaphragm Exercise – Most Important Muscle

When exercising your abdominal muscles, you will also be exercising your diaphragm, especially in the upward and downward pushing movements. Here is a special exercise for your diaphragm: *locate your diaphragm* by placing one hand at your waistline, then with the other hand hold the palm upward in front of your mouth. Now blow imaginary dust from the palm. Where you feel a strong muscular contraction when blowing, that's the location of **your diaphragm, the most important muscle you use when doing Bragg Super Power Breathing.**

4 Walk around your room on bare tiptoes, with your hands stretching up, reaching high over your head. Raise your diaphragm as high as your strength will allow, still breathing deeply. Feel it stretch chest and stomach muscles as you breathe deeply. Now bend over, drop head below heart, arms towards floor, then circle your arms in front of chest, compressing out every bit of toxic, carbon dioxide-laden air. Do this often, as it's a super lung cleanser and health builder.

It's a great habit to suck the oxygen-bearing fresh air deeply and slowly into your lungs. If you feel a little dizzy with the sudden oxygen stimulation, stop for a moment, then continue. *Begin by doing this diaphragm stretch – deep breathing exercise 5 times, gradually increasing to 10.* When you are able to do this exercise with ease, you are ready to start your Bragg Super Power Breathing Program (page 71).

Singing – Breathing Exercise

What is more elemental to singing than the breathing in and out of pure air into your hard-working lungs? Projecting sound and sustaining a note is hallmark of strong breathing muscles just as a lean, firm body is the sign of healthy, fit living. With singing, *(also whistling)* just as in breathing, the diaphragm and abdomen take lead roles and this exercise will help you master their use.

While standing up straight, feet 12 inches apart, place your left and right hand fingers on bottom ribs with thumbs gently probing below bottom rib. Now slowly draw in a full, deep diaphragmatic breath while feeling your abdominal movements with all fingers. Hold your breath for 5 seconds, now slowly exhale . . . but don't just "breathe out", instead, you should "sing out" the air. So, as you slowly let your breath out, softly sing a sustained note, as in "aa-hhh" or "oo-hhh". Note the abdominal movements with your fingers again. Repeat exercise 3 to 5 times. This helps you extend your control over the flow of sound and breath and helps you master your miracle breathing machinery.

Candle – Breathing Exercise

 In this version of the singing exercise, instead of holding your sides you hold a candle in front of your mouth. Again, slowly sing out your breath as evenly as possible – and thus exercise mastery of your breathing by controlling the candle flame.

Nature cannot be hastened. The bloom of a flower opens in its own proper time. – Paul Bruton

---

Diaphragmatic breathing is beneficial – it enhances circulatory function and relaxes muscles of ribs, chest and stomach. – Susan Smith Jones, Ph.D.

Little deeds of kindness, little words of love and thanks, help to make earth happy, like the Heaven above. – Julia A. F. Carney

Arm Pumping – Breathing Exercise

Stretching up spine, stand tall, legs relaxed with feet 12 inches apart. Drop arms down at sides. Now gradually pump arms up and down bird-style, breathing in through your mouth until your arms are up above your head. Grasp hands, stretch up, hold breath for 5 seconds. Now slowly breathe out as you bend down, relaxed, dropping arms and head below your heart. Repeat twice.

Controlled Deep Breathing For Super Oxygen

1 Enjoy this exercise before getting up in the morning and then repeat often during your day. It's also relaxing just before sleep. Count to yourself as you gently exhale and slowly inhale (vary breathing through the mouth and the nose). When you become more adept, then increase the count.

It's challenging to have breathing contests with your mate, family and friends to see who can take the deepest, slowest, longest breaths! This exercise will strengthen your lungs, chest and all muscles around your mid-waist. It also improves lung capacity and super breathing power as it gives firmer, trimmer waistline. This will help you learn to breathe in and out with control, varying breathing through the mouth and nose! When on walks pay attention to how long it takes to inhale and exhale. Ideally exhaling should be longer.

Diaphragmatic Panting Breathing Exercise: Super Oxygenator For Super Healthy Living

2 Raise your arms so that your ribs are separated. Rather than breathe as you normally would, pant while breathing. Pant until your diaphragm is tired. Your exhale panting should take about twice as long as your inhale panting. For example, if your inhale lasts for a count of 6, try to make your exhale last to 12. Do this exercise daily, especially before retiring. This helps re-oxygenate your entire body and remove the toxins from your system so you can enjoy a peaceful, restful and recharging sleep.

One-Breath Meditation Works Miracles

3 ATP (adenosine triphosphate) is a naturally occurring by-product of breathing that regulates physical action, thought and feeling. Dips in ATP levels can cause fatigue, aches and pains. The one-breath meditation exercise helps reverse the falling levels of important needed ATP.

1. *Sit in a comfortable chair and straighten up your spine, keeping shoulders back and relaxed.*

2. *Now inhale slowly and deeply, clear your mind completely. Relax shoulders and back. Imagine yourself in a secret garden, deeply drawing in peace and vitality from the oxygen rich air.*

3. *Hold your breath for a moment, then exhale slowly and fully, releasing all the tension from all your muscles and body.*

Use this one minute refresher at home, work and throughout the day as needed to refresh, restore and recharge your body, mind and soul – it works miracles!

Breathing Exercises During Pregnancy and Childbirth Benefits Mother and Baby

In natural childbirth classes (waterbirth, birthing chair, etc.) parents are taught certain breathing techniques, as Lamaze or Bradley, to help make childbirth easier and more comfortable. Visit webs: *www.lamazevideo.com, ecstaticbirth.com* and *www.informedbirth.com.* Mothers who practice the Bragg Super Breathing throughout their pregnancies have stronger muscles. This enhances their ability to make use of other breathing techniques and helps make the birthing process easier. This ensures that the mother and baby will have a healthier, happier, birthing experience. The primary benefits for the mother are a shortened recovery time and the ability to fully participate in the joyful process of her child's birth. For the baby, the primary benefit comes from the well-oxygenated blood the mother had been providing for the 9 months she carried the child in her womb. This oxygen helps prevent birth defects and helps ensure that the baby is born healthier and ready for a healthy, long life! To learn more about waterbirths, see website: *www.waterbirth.org.*

Chapter 11

Bragg Super Power Breathing Exercises

Faithfulness Counts Towards Super Health

The basic principle of Bragg Super Power Breathing is to fill the lungs to capacity with oxygen, then hold breath in, leaning forward, drop your head below your heart. This uses the force of gravity to infuse the head's cavities with oxygenated blood, which energizes the brain and helps maintain and create new brain cells (see page 16).

Every person who is interested in Super Health should take time each morning to do these Super Power Breathing Exercises. Take your present physical condition into consideration when you start on this program. Go slowly at first. Large parts of your lungs have probably been dormant for some time! It will take time to gradually open up these areas. Daily exercises will bring miracle results.

Make these exercises a daily habit, as much a part of your life as dressing, brushing your teeth and eating. The wonderful results obtained from faithfully following these breathing exercises and lifestyle will repay you abundantly with more health, energy, peace and longevity!

Love makes the world go 'round, and it's everlasting when it's given with caring, loving advice that will improve and enrich your life! This is why my father and I love sharing with you the health wisdoms which can be with you on your life's long happy journey. Our Bragg books on health, longevity and fitness go around the world spreading health and love! – Patricia Bragg, ND, PhD.

Nature, time and patience are the 3 greatest physicians. – Wise Irish Proverb

Accuse not nature, she hath done her part; now do thine!
– John Milton, Author, "Paradise Lost"

 Breathing only in the upper chest avoids the strong creative energies of the abdomen and sexual organs. Breathing only in the abdomen avoids the powerfully creative energies of the heart and throat. – Michael G. White

Exercise 1 – The Cleansing Breath

This is your Basic Super Power Breathing Exercise. All Super Power Breathing Exercises begin this way. Stand erect, feet about 15 to 18 inches apart, hands and arms relaxed at your sides (figure a). Raise your hands overhead (figure b). Now bend forward as far as possible – keeping your knees slightly bent and relaxed – exhaling at the same time through your mouth. Compress your chest and push upward with your diaphragm and abdominal muscles to expel all the stale air out of your lungs (figure c).

(a)   (b)   (c)   (d)   (e)

Now slowly inhale air through nose and mouth, pushing air downward with diaphragm and expanding your chest at its front and sides. Continue to draw in air to the full capacity of your lungs as you return to a standing position, while bringing your arms upward in a half-circle to the overhead position (figure d).

To complete the Cleansing Breath Exercise: As your hands reach the overhead position, then tighten your diaphragm and hold your breath for four or five seconds (mentally counting, *one thousand one, one thousand two,* etc.) while pulling your abdominal muscles back as if to pin your stomach to your backbone. Then exhale completely while bending forward, as in figure c & e. Now inhale as you return up as figure b and repeat exercise. Do this Cleansing Breath Exercise 5 times.

The quality of breath should be deep, graceful, easy and efficient. – Kenneth Cohen

Man is fully responsible for his nature and his choices. – Jean Paul Sartre

It's never too late to get into shape, but it does take daily perseverance.
– Dr. Thomas K. Cureton – Physical Fitness Pioneer, University of Illinois

72

Exercise 2 – The Super Power Brain Breath

Start by exhaling and inhaling as in Exercise 1. When your hands reach the overhead position, hold your breath (hold nose closed if necessary) and bend forward from the waist, knees bent, dropping your head below your heart, downward as far as possible. Continue to hold your breath to the count of 10 (mentally counting, *One thousand one, one thousand two*, etc.). This exercise allows the richly oxygenated blood to suffuse the pituitary gland on its way to reaching, refreshing and recharging every part of your brain for sharper thinking (work, school, etc.). This power breathing also helps cleanse the skull cavities (important and vital sinuses, ears, nose, eyes and mouth).

While holding your breath, now return to a standing position. Then bend forward, exhaling vigorously through the mouth. Slowly inhale as you return to starting standing position. Do this exercise 5 times at the beginning, gradually increasing to 10 repetitions.

NOTE: In these exercises, you may not be able to hold your breath for the full count at first. If you begin to feel dizzy, exhale and return to the standing position, dropping your arms to your sides and relax for a few minutes before continuing the exercise. You will gradually build your oxygen tolerance and be able to do the full count.

Health and intellect are two blessings of life. – Menander

Nothing transforms as much as changing from a negative to a positive attitude!

You are never too old to set another goal or to dream a new dream. – C.S. Lewis

73

Exercise 3 – The Super-Kidney Breath

Locate your kidneys on the lower back, just below the end of your rib cage near the waistline. Get the *feel* of them by placing your palms over this area, fingers and thumbs pointed downward. Use this position during the breath-holding part.

Exhale and inhale as at beginning of Exercise 1. As your hands reach the overhead position, tighten your diaphragm and pin your stomach to your backbone with your abdominal muscles, while holding your breath. Then firmly place your palms, with light pressure, over kidneys (on back below waist) relax knees and bend backward for a silent count of 10 (*One thousand one, two thousand two,* etc.). Still holding your breath, return to standing position. Then bend forward while exhaling vigorously through the mouth. (Use same precautions as in Exercise 2.) Slowly inhale as you return to the starting position. Do this exercise 5 times at the start, gradually increasing to 10.

Exercise 4 – For Easier Flowing Bowels

Do this exercise in the bathroom soon after rising each morning, and several times within an hour after eating. If you make this a habit, you will soon find you will have a bowel movement upon arising and an hour after eating. Taking a psyllium husk veg. cap after dinner works great!

Exhale and inhale as beginning Exercise 1. Now, holding breath, clasp hands in front and slowly lower yourself into relaxed squatting position while still holding your breath. Then strain for bowel movement for several seconds. Return to standing position and now by exhaling and inhaling as in previous exercises. Note: Squatting is natural way to have easy bowel movements. Children squat naturally. It opens up anal area more directly. Putting feet up on wastebasket or footstool when on toilet gives the same effect. Also stretch arms up above head so transverse colon will empty easier (page 182).

ELIMINATE THE "DRIBBLES" EXERCISE: To keep bladder and sphincter muscles tight and toned, urinate – stop – urinate – stop, 4 times, twice daily when voiding, especially after age of 40. This simple exercise works wonders for both men and women!

74

Exercise 5 – Filling the Lungs

This exercise is designed to get oxygen into the little-used air sacs at the bottom (apex) of the lungs, down near your waistline. Exhale and inhale as at the start of Exercise 1. But instead of returning the arms to the overhead position, relax them at your sides and bring your feet together, toes and heels touching. While holding your breath, bend to the right and reach toward the floor with the fingers of your right hand, at the same time bringing the left hand up to touch under the left armpit. Hold this position for a silent count of 10. Return to starting position and exhale and inhale as before. Now repeat the breath-holding position on left side. Reach toward floor with left hand while placing right hand under right armpit for count of 10. Repeat this exercise 5 to 10 times, alternating sides.

Exercise 6 – The Super Power Liver Cleansing Breath

Exhale and inhale as at the beginning of Exercise 1. Now bring feet together and clasp your fingers overhead, palms upward. Keep legs stiff from the hips down. Now holding a full breath, bend slowly to right side, then the left side, with as much stretch as possible. Now after doing left and right side stretches, return to starting position, but with feet apart. Next exhale with the usual forward bend, forcing all the old air out and then breathe in as you come up. Do 5 sets, gradually increasing to 10 repetitions of this liver cleansing exercise that promotes cleansing and circulation.

liver

Modern society lives in an unhealthy way that produces many over-worked livers. When we overeat, eat junk foods, and are exposed to environmental pollutants and stress, the liver becomes overworked and overloaded! – GlobalHealingCenter.com

Exercise 7 – Heart Strengthener

The purpose of this exercise is to expand the aorta, the main trunk of the arterial system which carries the blood from the heart after it has been oxygenated by Super Power Breathing. This exercise stimulates the circulation of blood in the heart, as well as the entire body, cardiovascular system, etc. It also helps recharge and increase the power of the respiratory system. This exercise also helps give relief to those who suffer from the feelings of suffocation and apprehension caused by asthma, angina pectoris, etc. (See Healthy Heart Habits page 182. Live a healthy lifestyle, plus drink 8 glasses of distilled water daily.)

This exercise starts with exhaling and inhaling as in the beginning of Exercise 1 (page 72), except that the arms are held forward at shoulder height (not overhead). When you return to the standing position, hold your breath – clasp your nose tightly with thumb and index finger so that no air escapes. Then pretend you are blowing your nose. You should feel some air pressure in your ears.

Now, with knees bent, bend over from the waist and gently bring your head down below your heart and midriff. Continue to hold your breath for a silent count of 10.

Return to the starting position and exhale and inhale in the usual Bragg Super Power Breathing manner (see page 72). Repeat this exercise 5 times, gradually increasing to 10 repetitions.

Coronary heart disease is due to a lack of oxygen received by the heart.
– Dr. Dean Ornish, Author of "Stress, Diet and Your Heart" (www.amazon.com)

Symptoms of heart failure reflect the diminished blood flow to all organs in the body, especially the lungs, kidneys, and liver. Such symptoms include shortness of breath, difficulty breathing when lying down and swelling in lower extremities or lower back. Take CoQ10 for a healthier heart. – LifeExtension.com

Always do what is right – despite any public opinions.

Cultivate Habit of Deep Breathing: *Diaphragmatic Breathing promotes a more relaxed state and makes the heart's job easier. Take a long, slow, deep breath right now! Visualize the air filling the lower part of your lungs. Do this for three minutes every hour during the day and notice the improvement.*

Chapter 12

Breathing Exercises to Enjoy For More Super Energy

The Bragg Super Power Breathing exercises are powerful for super health! Here are ways to add more variety for your enjoyment. Make some or all of these exercises a part of your daily health routine to give you more super vitality, health, creativity and fitness in your life.

Posture Breathing Exercise

The following activity is designed to correct bad posture habits, which are among the greatest impediments to proper breathing. Practice this activity several times a day at the job and at home. It will bring relief to your tired shoulders, spine and eyes, making you more alert and energized.

While you're sitting relaxed in a chair, then let your chin rest on your upper chest as you slowly lean forward, slowly exhaling. With eyes closed continue leaning until hands and elbows rest comfortably on your upper legs. After slowly exhaling in this position, sit upright quickly while sniffing in a full breath of fresh air through the nose. As you do this let your eyes open wide and then hold your full breath for 10 seconds (if necessary, first begin with holding for 5 second counts).

Take special note of how the sudden inhalation works to force your posture to healthy alignment as you sit up straight. After holding the inhaled breath, slowly release air through the mouth. Then close your eyes, lean forward and then repeat the exercise two more times.

Super Power Breathing for Fresh, New Air

Because the majority of people don't use their full lungs' capacity, the following exercise is designed to get new air into the forgotten, unused regions of the lungs. Practice moderately at first, but with greater frequency as your lungs will soon become healthier and stronger!

Comfortably sit or stand and now inhale slowly through the nose a complete, deep diaphragmatic breath. As you do this let your head be comfortably lifted backwards until it has come to rest as far back as it can without strain. After holding this position and your breath for 3 to 5 seconds, slowly exhale through closed teeth as your head moves forward to the starting position. As you exhale (there should be a hissing noise as the air is forced between the teeth) concentrate on expelling all of the old air out of your lungs. Repeat this exercise several times. It's particularly suitable to pre-aerobic warm-ups because it will prepare the lungs for super oxygenation.

Rejuvenation Breathing Exercise

When areas of the lungs have remained unused, the pathways can become narrowed or even closed. This breathing exercise helps rejuvenate the lungs by opening up the passageways to the lungs' neglected areas! Do this activity moderately and gently at first. But as your lungs become healthier and stronger, increase the frequency and enjoy the force of your breathing exertion.

While standing, take in a deep, full diaphragmatic breath and lift your chin up slightly. Once you have taken in the full breath, hold it in and stand still. Then raise your bent arms chest high and with closed fists gently pound your upper chest area (still holding your breath) in gorilla style. Also pound your rib areas and the lower lung region. Do this for as long as you can comfortably hold your breath. As you exhale, knees relaxed, bend head down below heart and exhale as much old air as possible from your lungs. Repeat this exercise several times.

With a full breath swelling your lungs, this gentle pounding (patting) exercise opens up those passageways that haven't carried air for a long time. The more passages you have available to move air through your lungs and into your blood, the more energy and vitality and the better health and fitness you will experience.

To desire to be healthy is important part of being healthy.
– Seneca, Roman Philosopher, 65 AD

Exercise to Increase Lungs' Air Space

This breathing exercise helps you make use of your lungs' maximum breathing capacity in a comfortable and gentle manner. Practice several times a day to enjoy more energy and fitness on the job and at home.

While standing, knees relaxed, bend over and exhale completely all the old stale air. You can help your lungs expel (push out) the air by pulling in your belly muscles, forcing your stomach inwards towards your spine. Now stand straight, slowly inhale, filling your lungs to full capacity and hold your breath for 20 seconds (if 20 seconds is not possible, set a challenging, non-painful goal). As you count, slowly stretch your arms up over your head. This will stretch your lungs, maximizing their air space. When you have completed your breath holding pattern, relax and bend down and exhale air slowly. Do this 2 or 3 more times and increase as desired.

Exercise for A Flexible, Youthful Rib Cage

As with the preceding exercise, this maximizes the body's spatial capacity for breathing. The previous exercise works on increasing the lungs' air holding capacity. This exercise works on the space your rib cage can make available for your lungs to expand.

While standing, exhale completely with arms at your sides. Slowly inhale, filling your lungs to capacity and hold your breath for 20 seconds. As you count place your palms on your hips with your thumbs forward and your pinkie fingers touching each other at your lower spine.

Now pull elbows backward far as possible while holding your breath. Then exhale slowly moving arms down to sides. Repeat 2 or 3 times. This exercise helps keep the rib area flexible, so to maximize your air lung space.

A strong body makes a strong mind! – Thomas Jefferson, 3rd U.S. President, 1801-1809

We must always change, renew, rejuvenate ourselves; otherwise, we harden. – Johann W. Goethe

Exercise To Maximize Chest Area

This exercise will also help you maximize the available chest and rib cage area for your lungs to expand and take in more air. Practice several times daily along with the other air capacity increasing exercises.

Starting position – stand with your arms at sides, inhale deeply through the nose, then while holding your breath for 5 seconds, extend arms forward, now clasp hands together and stretch hands up, high above your head, exhaling quickly and fully through your mouth. Naturally your upper chest will move upward with this high up stretch. Now return to starting position and repeat 2 or 3 times.

Breathing Exercise for Lower Lungs

The lungs' lower regions are the most distant from your windpipe, and the most dependent on the breathing activity of the diaphragm. As a result, the lungs' lower regions are the most likely areas to suffer disuse. This important exercise is designed to bring more air to these under-used areas of the lungs.

While lying on the floor on an exercise/foam pad, concentrate on your lower lungs. Put tip of index finger just below your belly button and consider this spot the center of your lower lungs. Slowly inhale through the nose a full and total breath, concentrating on filling the lung area beneath your finger first. With practice you will soon find that you can easily target your breathing in this way. As you inhale fill your lower lungs first (beneath finger), moving to your familiar upper lungs last.

After a few days of practice your skill level in this exercise will noticeably increase and you will find it easy to aim your breathing to different regions of your lungs. Once you have this ability, practice this exercise while standing or lying down, at home or at work. You will find that it is both soothing and invigorating, and suitable both for before sleep and for energy when tired.

Nerve Force contains much of its power in the breath. – Yoga Teachings

Deep, Slow Breathing
Promotes Relaxed, Peaceful Sleep

Millions worldwide suffer from insomnia – bad sleep and bad sleeping habits. Preparing sensibly for a good night's rest – ventilated room, firm mattress with memory 2" foam topper – is one of the easiest ways to improve your ability to sleep well (for more tips see pages 97-98). The following deep breathing exercise relaxes the body and reduces mental stress to prepare for a peaceful, recharging sleep so vital to your health and well-being!

Lie in bed on your back with hands at your sides, palms down. Close your eyes and quiet your mind as you slowly inhale through your nose to fill your lower lungs first. As you inhale, raise your arms in a slow circling motion up over your head. Aim to complete your inhalation just as your 2 thumbs touch each other, with arms then resting behind your head. Hold this breath for 10-15 seconds. Exhale slowly through mouth as you reverse your arm circling motion, bringing arms back to starting position at sides. Repeat this exercise several times or until relaxed and drowsy.

Another breathing techniques you may try, when you first get into bed: 1) Take a deep breath. 2) Breathe in through your nose and visualize the air moving down to your stomach. 3) As you breathe in again silently count to four. 4) Purse your lips as you exhale slowly. 5) This time count silently to eight. 6) Repeat this process 6-10 times.

The results of this breathing technique are immediate. You will feel your shoulders and arms relaxing. Your chest will feel less constricted and you will feel less stress and tension! The goal is to relax your mind and let your body unwind and surrender to peaceful sleep.

For Insomnia and Nervous Tension use these Herbs:

Chamomile oil: *put in bath water (5-6 drops) to soothe nerves, dilute to 2% to make excellent massage oil. Chamomile tea, 2-3 times daily.*

Passion Flower: *for insomnia due to worry, overwork or nervous exhaustion. Excellent sedative with no side effects. Drink tea 3 times a day.*

Valerian: *for insomnia or if having hard time falling asleep helps reduce night wakings with no negative effects. Drink Valerian tea as needed.*

Fast Help for Panicky, Stressful Moments

Stress and fear tightens the entire body, especially the breathing muscles. Learn to relax and loosen the tightened muscles and panic and tensions will melt away.

These simple-to-do exercises will bring fast relief:

- Concentrate breathing in deeply and slowly through mouth, then blow out slowly all stress and tension.
- Wait! Don't breathe for a few seconds. While breath is out, force stomach muscles in and out 4 times.
- Slow shoulder rolls to ears – then roll shoulders back, down and around, then reverse rolls. Do 5 times.

You will soon be more relaxed and peaceful.

For a nervous stomach, do this finger acupressure:

Firmly press, massage skin between thumb and forefinger. This helps for car and plane sickness and a nervous stomach. Life is a journey of choices, now relax, be healthy, happy, peaceful and enjoy your healthy lifestyle and count all your blessings!

Try these Ten Great No-Calorie Stress Busters:

1. Turn on your favorite music and dance.
2. Enroll in a yoga class, or take tai chi, chi gong, Pilates or enjoy a stretching class.
3. Call a good friend and have some laughs.
4. Read inspiring Bragg books and health magazines.
5. Take hot herbal bubble bath or Bragg Vinegar ($1/2$ cup) bath.
6. Go to the gym or take a brisk fresh air health walk.
7. Get a massage – best at your home when possible.
8. Write and release your feelings in your daily journal.
9. Watch an inspiring movie, comedy or travelogue.
10. Close your eyes, relax, do 'yoga breathing' – breathe in slowly through nose, letting air fill lungs completely down to the diaphragm. Hold in briefly, then exhale through the mouth slowly. See: *HealthAndYoga.com.*

Breath is the spirit of life, the concentrated power or essence of physical being.
– Andrew Weil • www.BreathMastery.com

Chapter 13

Common Respiratory Ailments & Diseases

Breathing difficulties can come on suddenly or be a warning of a disease in the body! Breathing problems include pain, discomfort or any difficulty that interferes with the normal, natural cycle of easily inhaling and exhaling air. Respiratory diseases are becoming more common worldwide, particularly in industrialized countries like U.S. and China. Air pollution, cigarette smoke and congested living conditions are main problems.

Here's a list of some common breathing ailments:

- ● *Asthma:* A condition where airways are constricted, making breathing difficult. See pages: 85-89 for more health info on prevention and treatment of Asthma.

- ● *Bronchitis:* Inflammation of bronchial tubes, the airways that carry air to your lungs. It causes a cough that often brings up mucus, as well as shortness of breath, wheezing and chest tightness. See pages 90-91 for more info.

- ● *Chronic Obstructive Pulmonary Disease (COPD):* Progressive disease that makes it hard to breathe. Can cause coughing that produces large amounts of mucus, wheezing, shortness of breath and chest tightness. Cigarette smoking is leading cause of COPD. Long term exposure to other lung irritants – air pollution, chemical fumes or dust also may contribute to COPD. See pages 91-92 for more info.

- ● *Dyspnea:* Shortness of Breath – feeling like you cannot get enough air. You may experience shortness of breath just once or have recurring episodes. Very strenuous exercise, extreme temperatures, obesity and high altitude can cause Dyspnea in healthy person. Besides these, shortness of breath is likely a sign of a medical problem. **If you have unexplained shortness of breath, do see doctor as soon as possible!**

Alpha-1 Antitrypsin Deficiency: *An inherited disorder that may cause serious lung disease. The body does not make enough alpha-1 antitrypsin a protein in the blood that protects lungs from inflammation caused by infection and inhaled irritants as tobacco smoke, etc. Most common signs and symptoms caused by Alpha-1 is shortness of breath, wheezing, chronic bronchitis, chest cold, and allergies.* – Alpha-1Foundation.org

- **Emphysema:** Chronic lung disease, often caused by exposure to toxic chemicals or long-term exposure to tobacco smoke. Emphysema gradually damages the air sacs in lungs, making you progressively more short of breath. Symptoms are shortness of breath on exertion and hyperventilation (see info on COPD page 91-92).

- **Hyperventilation:** Rapid or deep breathing that can occur with anxiety or panic. *Treatment:* The goal is to raise carbon dioxide level in your blood, which helps end your symptoms. Do this old-fashioned remedy – breathe into paper bag for 3 minutes, it helps to restore carbon dioxide/oxygen levels in the lungs.

- **Pneumonia:** Common lung infections caused by bacteria, virus, fungi or diet. Symptoms can vary from mild to severe. *Prevention:* Frequently wash hands as flu can lead to pneumonia. Live the Bragg Healthy Lifestyle including a healthy diet (see page 39) and getting ample sleep. *Treatment:* Depends on cause of pneumonia, how severe symptoms are and your age and overall health.

- **Respiratory Distress Syndrome (RDS):** condition where body is not receiving enough oxygen from the lungs. Injuries, accidents, war injuries, infections or other conditions cause fluid to accumulate in air sacs. Then, fluid and proteins leak out from capillaries into alveoli, making whole lungs stiff. This prevents lungs from working properly. They cannot fill up with air in a normal way, neither can they get rid of carbon dioxide effectively. The signs for Respiratory Distress is: dizziness, shortness of breath, fatigue and low blood pressure. *Treatment:* patients are placed in ICU and put on air ventilator. The No. 1 priority is to raise your blood oxygen levels.

- **Sleep Apnea:** Common respiratory disorder that causes you to stop breathing briefly while you sleep. Sleep apnea can be treated. For more info see pages 102-104.

The average human inhales 3,000 gallons of air daily. Unfortunately millions breathe contaminated, toxic and sick air in homes, offices, work places, cities, and airplanes, etc.

Gently forced into action, most lungs will slowly rebuild themselves.

Create the kind of self you will be happy to live with all your life. – Foster C. McClellan

Prevention Methods for Breathing Problems:

- Avoid all tobacco smoke, smog, toxic vapors, etc.
- Exercise regularly – brisk healthy walking is great fun
- Avoid pollens, dust, molds, and other allergens
- Live the Bragg Healthy Lifestyle including: maintaining faithfully a healthy diet and a normal healthy weight
- Wash hands with perfume-free soap frequently
- Wear a mask when working around dust, chemicals, etc.

Millions of Americans Suffer with Asthma

Today nearly 25 million Americans suffer from asthma, 7.1 million are under the age of 18. Asthma accounts for 1.8 million emergency room visits and 12.8 million doctor visits a year. It's one of the great maladies of our polluted, poisoned age, costing $19.7 billion yearly. Five thousand Americans die from asthma yearly, sadly 14 every day.

Even in hospital emergency rooms with all that modern technology and pharmacological medicine they offer, more people are dying of asthma. In one New York City emergency room alone, last year 22 children died of asthma attacks.

Asthma is a reversible obstructive lung disease, caused by increased reaction of the airways to various stimuli. It is a chronic inflammatory condition with serious acute exacerbations. Asthma can be a life-threatening disease if not managed! Daily control is vital to living an active, productive, healthy life towards eliminating asthma.

Asthma breathing problems usually happen in short "episodes" or "attacks", but the inflammation underlying asthma is continuous. An asthma attack occurs when muscles surrounding the airway contract, narrowing air passages that are chronically swollen and inflamed. During an attack, the mucus fills the airway like a plug. When the victim breathes in, the air slides around the mucus obstructions. When the victim tries to exhale, the mucus plugs the airway, stopping flow of air out of lungs. Some trigger for asthma attacks are: Tobacco Smoke, Vapors, Dust, Air Pollution, Mites, Cockroach Allergen, Pets, Mold, Smoke from Burning Wood, Sinus Infections, Food Allergies (milk etc. see pages 39-40), Burning Incense, High Humidity.

Asthma and Toxic Allergy Triggers

Those with asthma should be wise and cautious of the triggers that cause attacks. Some triggers are food additives, aspirin, MSG and sulfites. In your home mold grows on shower curtains, bathtubs, tiles, etc. Dust mites favorite areas are blankets, pillows, carpets, stuffed toys, etc. Asthma can be triggered by smoke from the burning end of a cigarette or second hand smoke. Please don't smoke or allow others to smoke in home! Cockroach body parts and droppings may trigger asthma attacks. Cats and dogs dander are triggers. Nitrogen Dioxide gas can irritate eyes, nose, throat and may cause shortness of breath. This gas comes from appliances that burn gas, wood and kerosene, such as BBQ's, fireplaces and car exhaust. Chemical irritants and fragrances (buy only odor-free) can also be triggers! These are found in soaps, detergents, fabric softeners, cleaners, perfumes, aftershaves, colognes, deodorants, hairsprays, mothballs, candles, air fresheners, etc.

Gardenburger Creator Thanks Bragg Books
Cured His Asthma in a Month

Patricia with Paul Wenner

Paul Wenner, the *Gardenburger* Creator, says his early years as a youth with asthma were so bad he would stand at the window praying to breathe through the night and stay alive! A miracle happened when as a teenager he read Bragg Books on *Fasting, Breathing,* and *Healthy Lifestyle* and his years of asthma were cured in only one month! Paul became so inspired he wanted to be a Health Crusader like Paul Bragg and daughter Patricia – and Paul Wenner has! *Now Gardenburgers are sold worldwide. www.gardenburger.com*

After years of asthma, in a month I could breathe normally for first time in my life. It was a miracle! I thank Paul Bragg & Patricia for Bragg Fasting & Breathing Books.
– Paul Wenner, Creator of Gardenburger, Author, "Garden Cuisine"

More Americans than ever before say they are suffering from asthma. It is one of America's most common and costly diseases! – www.aafa.org

Treating Asthma Naturally Brings Results!

Famous Dr. Andrew Weil, stated in his Self Healing Letter, "*I have seen asthma disappear completely in response to major diet shifts such as eliminating sugar, milk products and switching to a healthy vegetarian regime.*" Johns Hopkins Hospital Studies and others suggest those who monitored their diets, low in meat, no milk and no additives, were less likely to have asthma problems. Sadly, most doctors believe erroneously there is no cure for asthma. Asthma attacks can be life-threatening. For short-term acute asthma help, bronchodilating drugs (often addictive with side effects) are at times necessary until breathing improves. There are natural remedies that, while not substitutes for bronchodilators, may help manage acute asthma episodes until breathing improves.

Butterbur Root: Studies have shown that patients who treated their asthma with butterbur in addition to prescribed steroid experienced much more freedom of air flow than those who treated with inhaled steroids alone. Make sure you get the certified PA-free product.

Ginkgo Biloba: has also been used to help patients deal with asthma. This herbal extract helps to block a compound known as PAF, or platelet activating factor, which plays a large role in the flare-ups of asthma symptoms.

Lobelia: is used by many naturopathic physicians to treat asthma. Keep on hand – mixture combining three parts tincture of lobelia with one part tincture of capsicum (red pepper). At start of asthmatic attack, take 5-10 drops of mixture in distilled water. As needed repeat every 30-60 minutes up to 4 times for total of 3 or 4 doses.

Eucalyptus Oil: Pure eucalyptus oil is an effective treatment for asthma symptoms because of its decongestant properties. Put 2-3 drops of eucalyptus oil in a pot of boiling water and deeply breathe in the steam.

---

*If using inhalers now – try medication called **Advair Diskus** that is giving relief to asthma suffers. Used daily it works as a preventative instead of an emergency asthma inhaler. For people who use a steroid inhaler multiple times daily, this may help bring permanent relief from having to use inhalers as often! We hope those who have breathing problems will soon be improved like Paul Wenner, that they will have less need for medication!*

For Long Term Control & Prevention of Asthma

- Decrease protein to 10% of daily caloric intake or even better replace animal protein with plant based proteins.

- Eliminate milk and milk products, substituting other calcium sources, such as soy, rice or almond milk.

- Eat organically grown fruits and vegetables.

- Eliminate polyunsaturated vegetable oils, margarine, vegetable shortening, all partially hydrogenated oils that might contain trans-fatty acids, and all foods that contain trans-fatty acids, such as deep-fried foods.

- Use Bragg Extra-Virgin Olive Oil as your main fat.

- Increase intake of omega-3's (flaxseeds and walnuts).

- Always drink plenty of distilled water to keep your respiratory tract secretions more fluid.

- Experiment with eliminating (one at a time) wheat (white flour), corn, soy and sugar for 6-8 weeks to see if the condition improves (keep daily journal – page 151).

- Eat ginger and turmeric for anti-inflammatory effects.

- Have manipulative work done on the chest to break up restrictive patterns in nerves and muscles that develop in chronic asthma. Best systems for this is Chest Tapping and Rolfing, a form of deep-tissue massage (see page 207).

- Minimize contact with respiratory irritants, such as smoke, dust, molds, and volatile organic compounds (VOC). Remove sources of offending materials from your home or office, install a good air filtration system. Experiment with living in other locations: in high mountains, the desert, or near the seacoast. Asthma may improve greatly with a change of climate.

- In adults, GERDs maybe an underlying asthma cause. In such cases, successful Bragg ACV treatment of digestive problems often helps clear up the asthma.

- Experiment with traditional Chinese Medicine and Ayurvedic Medicines. These systems are sometimes able to offer significant help through more specific dietary adjustments and herbal treatments.

Info from Dr. Andrew Weil an American medical doctor, naturopath, and writer on holistic health • DrWeil.com

Heimlich Maneuver Helps Asthma Attacks

There is hope for victims of asthma attacks. Our friends Dr. Henry Heimlich and his wife and author Jane Murray Heimlich (*daughter of famous dancing Arthur Murray*) are Health Crusaders, helping save lives worldwide! This versatile Heimlich Maneuver is life-saving for more than just choking victims! The Heimlich Institute (*deaconess-healthcare.com/Heimlich_Institute*) is currently teaching asthma patients how to push up on their own diaphragm (more gently than in cases of choking) to help expel trapped air and clear bronchials of mucus plugs. As Dr. Heimlich explains, *"We started receiving calls from people who had suffered severe, almost deadly asthma attacks."* He says, *"The people who were with them didn't have any idea what to do. They just tried Heimlich Maneuver and immediately, a miracle happened, the asthma attack stopped."*

Try the following technique for relief of asthma attack. Someone close to you should learn the Heimlich Maneuver, because it's a little difficult to do it for yourself. Stand behind the person having the attack, wrap your arms around the torso in a hug, and then, using both hands, lift the entire tummy and diaphragm upward, as if you were trying to push it up under ribs and breastbone, then apply Heimlich. This Heimlich Maneuver is similar for a choking person, read pages 200-203. When it's performed on asthmatics, the Heimlich Maneuver need only be done very gently because you are expelling mucus and trapped air – not a stuck, solid object, food, etc. or lungs full of water.

When they can breathe easily again, have them get down on their hands and knees, straddle them and repeat process. This technique helps the diaphragm return to its normal, healthy position easily. If the attack is severe and this technique doesn't work, be sure to quickly follow up with medical emergency help. Studies show applying this procedure on a regular basis keeps lungs free of mucus that can plug up the airway and bring on an asthma attack.

Studies reveal children who are overweight are 1.16 times more likely to develop asthma compared with children of normal weight. It is worse for moderately obese children – 1.23 times more likely to develop asthma. Obese children are 1.37 times more at risk, with more severe type of asthma. The CDC has stated that there are currently 7.1 million children in US suffering from asthma.

What is Bronchitis?

Bronchitis is the inflammation of mucus membranes of the main air passages of the lungs (the bronchial tree comprising the bronchi and the bronchioles). It causes congestion in the chest, cough, difficulty in breathing and chest tightness. Acute Bronchitis is generally caused by a lung infection, 90% of which are viral in origin. Most Americans with a sore throat or bronchitis are prescribed antibiotics even though just a fraction stand to benefit from them. Almost all sore throats are caused by viruses . . . "so an antibiotic is not going to help and it has a very real chance of hurting you," says Dr. Jeffrey Linder, Research for Brigham and Women's Hospital in Boston*.

Home Remedies to Help Cure Bronchitis

Instead of using antibiotics, here are a few home remedies that come in handy to anyone suffering from bronchitis or any other similar respiratory ailment. Try these remedies during the early stages and see results.

- Eating hot, spicy foods like chilli peppers, helps thin the mucus in your lungs and helps to drain your phlegm.

- Inhaling steam aids in loosening the secretions of the lungs, which drains phlegm. Take hot shower or breathe in steam from hot boiling water with Bragg Apple Cider Vinegar or Oil of Oregano added (see page 33). Also try eucalyptus, lavender or peppermint oils (see page 38).

- Avoid alcohol, caffeinated drinks, and instead drink plenty of purified water or make Bragg Vinegar Drink (page 149).

- Mix half teaspoon honey with 2 powdered cloves and pinch of pepper – cures burning sensation in the chest and relieves congestion, leading to better breathing.

- Try mixture of ground linseed/flaxseed and sesame seeds laced with honey. Helps relieve respiratory problems.

*Antibiotics can have bad side effects, including: stomach pain, yeast infections and severe diarrhea. They can also cause drug-resistant germs – which means future infections could be harder to treat (also beware of antibacterial soaps). Antibiotics should only be prescribed if you have strep throat, which is caused by bacteria that could be killed with antibiotics. – Reuters.com

- Mix crushed almonds in a glass of freshly squeezed orange juice. Regular use of this can help quell respiratory troubles. Besides Vitamin C supplements and fresh fruit juices helps to fight respiratory viruses.
- Boil a few leaves of basil in water and drink it.
- Ginger is a very good remedy for most of the respiratory disorders. Make a tea by adding half teaspoon of freshly grated ginger, ground cloves and ground black pepper and allow to boil. You can sweeten it with honey to help build immunity against diseases and allergies.
- Drink one teaspoon raw onion juice in morning, great remedy for bronchitis and other respiratory infections.

About Chronic Obstructive Pulmonary Disease

In the US the term "COPD" includes two main conditions – *emphysema* and *chronic bronchitis*. Chronic bronchitis is an inflammation of the lining of your bronchial tubes, which carry air to and from your lungs. Emphysema occurs when the air sacs (alveoli) at the end of the smallest air passages (bronchioles) in the lungs are gradually destroyed. Most people who have COPD have both emphysema and chronic bronchitis. Thus, the general term "COPD" is more accurate.

COPD is a major cause of disability and is the 3rd leading cause of death in US. Currently, millions of people (6.3% of population) are diagnosed or have COPD. The main cause of COPD is tobacco smoking! Other irritants can cause COPD, including cigar smoke, secondhand smoke, pipe smoke, air pollution and workplace exposure to dust, smoke or fumes. COPD has no cure and doctors don't know how to reverse the damage. However, treatments and lifestyle changes can help you feel better and stay more active and slow the progress of the disease. Info from *www.nhlbi.nih.gov* and *www.mayoclinic.org*

*Studies show that using **Mullein** may help in treating COPD. Laboratory results show that mullein kills viruses on contact in test tubes, and may boost effectiveness of some medications that treat influenza. It can help break up phlegm and soothe irritated mucus membranes. Mullein is available as liquid or dried extract. You can make mullein tea by adding 1-2 tsps. of dried leaves and flowers to 1 cup boiling water and steep for 10 minutes. – LiveStrong.com*

COPD Natural Remedies and Treatments

Quit Smoking: According to American Thoracic Society (ATS), about 90% of people with COPD get the disease from smoking. Quitting is the most important lifestyle change you can make to ease COPD symptoms. Prolonged chronic asthma can progress into lung destructing emphysema.

Stay Active: Staying physically active is the second most important thing you can do at home to help manage symptoms of COPD. According to Mayo Clinic, regular exercise can actually strengthen your respiratory muscles, improve your breathing and your overall strength and endurance. Try brisk walking, jogging, gardening, golfing, tennis or even shopping (see page 186-187).

Eat Right: Eating healthy foods and maintaining a proper weight can significantly help improve breathing. For more info on eating a healthy diet see pages 125-128.

Control Breathing: Breathing exercises and relaxation techniques can help you breathe more efficiently throughout the day. See Bragg Super Power Breathing Exercises on pages 71-81. These breathing exercises increase your blood oxygen levels and help reduce shortness of breath.

Stay Hydrated: drink plenty of purified water and fruit juices. Use humidifier to keep airways clear of mucus.

Protect Yourself: When you have COPD, it's important to avoid situations that can aggravate your symptoms. Cold air can trigger bronchospasm, a sudden constriction in the muscles of airway walls that leads to shortness of breath! Respiratory infections can cause COPD symptoms to worsen, so wise to stay away from crowds if possible.

Take Care of Your Emotions: The changes in your life caused by COPD and its symptoms may cause you to experience some difficult emotions. Grief, anger, anxiety, and depression are all normal responses to chronic illness.

Reduce Stress: Stress can exacerbate COPD symptoms like shortness of breath, so it's important to manage the level of stress in your life! Take some time each day to unwind, both physically and mentally. You can relax by napping, listening to soothing music, reading quietly, or doing something that you find enjoyable and soothing.

Deep Breathing and Bragg Healthy Lifestyle Can Revitalize Lungs with More Oxygen

Prolonged chronic asthma can often progress into lung destructing emphysema and COPD. This causes air sacs to become so distended with trapped stale air they lose elasticity, and can slowly suffocate. Bragg Super Power Breathing can't restore destroyed tissue, but helps salvage and revitalize the rest of the lungs! The life-giving inflow of oxygen acts as a natural decongestant and gradually cleans out bronchioles and bronchial tubes! This helps remove toxic carbon dioxide and other waste from air sacs and lung tissues. This cleansing and opening-up of lungs helps revitalize every possible cell with more oxygen and nutrients!

Respiratory ailment victims have gained permanent relief by following The Bragg Healthy Lifestyle and eliminating all milk products, ice cream, yogurt, cheese, butter, etc., along with fasting for 24 hour period weekly and eating a healthy vegetarian live foods diet. It's absolutely essential you eliminate all cow's milk and its products from your diet, as these produce mucus and sickness!

Do Bragg Super Power Breathing exercises (pages 71-81), gradually increase walks and exercise. Take vitamin C and E, CoQ10 and Braggzyme (see pages 152, 155, 157-158); they promote lung tissue healing and help reduce inflammatory and bronchial wall swelling. Read page 38 for herbs and supplements. Make sure to eat healthy diet – organic fruits and vegetables, nuts, seeds, whole grains, beans, legumes, etc. (see pages 125-128). Drink 8 glasses of purified/distilled water daily, keeps you hydrated. Make sure you get sufficient sleep – at least 8 hours nightly (see pages 95-98). Get plenty of gentle sunshine and fresh air daily (see pages 195-198). For more info on The Bragg Healthy Lifestyle please read Bragg Books: *Healthy Lifestyle*, *Miracle of Fasting*, *Apple Cider Vinegar*, and *Water-Shocking Truth*.

Next time you toss an orange peel, don't! Grate, sprinkle on foods. Organic orange peels are rich powerful flavonoid antioxidants that reduce oxidative damage and fight free radicals! Plus are loaded with natural histamine – a suppressing compound that can help expel congestion associated with bronchitis, colds and flu. Helps keep lungs cleansed. – NaturalNews.com

Important Self-Health Care for Healthy Lungs

Because standard drugs are suppressive in nature, they tend to perpetuate asthma and reduce the chance that it will disappear on its own – especially in children. Try these natural self-care measures to prevent attacks, improve lungs health and lessen the need for any drugs.

• **Use a peak-flow meter,** a hand-held device that you can blow into to measure the amount of air in your lungs.

• **Reduce asthma and respiratory triggers** by learning causes. Try to eliminate all destructive triggers from your life.

• **Drink 8-10 glasses of purified/distilled water daily,** to help keep respiratory-tract secretions moist and fluid. Drinking plenty of water speeds process of eliminating irritants and toxins from the body. Avoid dehydration!

• **Supplement your diet daily with 3,000 mg. vitamin C.**

• **Say "no" to milk & dairy products** which increases mucus that worsens asthma and allergies! Visit: *NotMilk.com*

• **Change your diet.** Food allergies (pages 39-40) trigger chronic asthma attacks and respiratory-breathing problems.

• **Be manipulated.** Go to Chiropractor or Osteopath and have them check for any restrictions in back, neck, chest and diaphragm areas. A skilled practitioner can free them up. When needed this can help promote healing and health.

• **Exercise wisely.** Warm up slowly with stretching and breathing exercises (at least 10-15 minutes). Don't walk or jog within 50 feet of a heavy traffic road (car fumes are toxic). Enjoy parks with lawns, trees and fresh clean air.

• **Clear the air.** Use HEPA filters (page 119) in whole room areas or entire house filter system and also use in your car.

• **Hang some plants** (Spider plants, Boston ferns, English Ivy, etc.) in your house, work, office, etc. Plants absorb toxic vapors and gases that help purify the air for your lungs.

• **Relax.** Do breathing exercises and rest (pgs. 71-81, 163-168).

• **Consider healing healthy alternatives** (pages 205-208). Example: a young asthmatic patient was so improved after two months of a Ayurvedic health treatment that he dispensed with most of his medication (pages 46-47).

Chapter 14

Sleeping & Snoring Problems

America's National "Sleep Debt"

The National Sleep Foundation poll taken recently discovered that a whopping 67% of American adults have a sleeping problem and that over one-third (37%), are so sleepy during the daytime that their daily activities are interfered with. Over the past 100 years, we've reduced our average sleep time by 20% and, over the last 25 years, added an additional month to our annual work/commute time. Our national "sleep debt" is rising and while our society has changed, our physical bodies and needs have not! We are paying dearly for such unhealthy "progress"! Visit their informative website: *www.SleepFoundation.org.*

Are You Getting Enough Sleep Lately?

The odds are you are not getting sufficient sleep. American adults presently average 7 hours nightly. While everyone's sleep needs vary, most scientific research indicates that we require 8 hours of sleep nightly. Few are lucky enough to enjoy 5 to 6 hours of sound sleep and still perform well at work. To just get "caught up," a full ten hours of rest, plus naps are frequently called for!!!

First make a clear choice about how you wish to spend the 30-45 minutes that precede your actual going to bed. Avoid a rush to "get things ready for tomorrow" or to catch up on tasks not completed during the day. This is a time to relax and rest your body and mind. Try an aroma herbal bath or a self-massage (Bragg Olive Oil) while showering, one hour before bed – it's so relaxing. Enjoy a warm soothing Bragg Apple Cider Vinegar drink with cinnamon and honey (recipe on page 149) or a Lemon Balm or Sleepytime herbal tea before bedtime. Lemon Balm, whose scientific name is *melissa officinalis,* is a soothing plant with both nervine and antiseptic, relaxing natural qualities. It's a member of the peppermint and spearmint family and is grown worldwide. When flowering it has a lemon fragrance – a perfume delight.

Good Sleep is Cornerstone of Good Health

Eight hours nightly is the optimal amount of sleep for most adults! Science has established that a sleep deficit can have serious, far reaching effects on your health!

Interrupted or Lack of Proper Sleep Can:

- Dramatically weaken your immune system
- Accelerate tumor growth with severe sleep dysfunctions
- Cause a pre-diabetic state, making you feel hungry and then you over fuel your body causing obesity
- Seriously impair your memory. Even a single night of poor sleep (4-6 hours) can impact ability to think clearly
- Impair your performance on physical or mental tasks
- Can also increase stress-related disorders including: Heart Disease, Stomach Ulcers, Constipation, Mood Disorders, Personality Upsets and Depression

Healthful Tips for Sound, Recharging Sleep
Excerpts from Dr. Mercola – www.mercola.com

The good news is there are many natural techniques you can learn to restore your "sleep health". Whether you have difficulty falling asleep or feel inadequately rested when waking up, you can find some relief from the tips below:

• **Sleep in complete darkness.** Even the tiniest bit of light in the room can disrupt your internal clock and your pineal gland's production of melatonin and serotonin. Little bits of light pass directly through your optic nerve to your hypothalamus, which controls your biological clock. Light signals your brain that it's time to wake up and starts preparing your body for ACTION!!!

• **Wear an eye mask to block out light.** It is not always easy to block out every stream of light using curtains or blinds.

The average person spends about 24 years of a 78 year lifespan asleep.

A recharging, peaceful good night sleep is vitally important!

Your word is a lamp to my feet and a light to my path. – Psalm 119:105

• **Keep bedroom lower temp 60-65°F best for sleeping.** Scientists believe cooler bedroom is most conducive to sleep since it mimics body's natural temperature drop.

• **Check bedroom for Electro-Magnetic Fields** (EMFs). EMF's can disrupt pineal gland and production of melatonin and serotonin. To check this you will need a gauss meter (Radio Shack or check web: *LessEMF.com/gauss.html*). Before going to bed unplug any phones, clocks or radios near bed. I do even when in hotels – PB! (see below)

• **Move alarm clocks and other electric devices away from your bed.** It will only add to your worry when you stare at it all night – 2 am – 3 am – 4:30 am. Prior to use of electricity, people would go to bed shortly after sundown and then rise with the sun as most animals do. Wise Mother Nature intended this for humans as well.

• **Get to bed as early as possible.** Your body recharges between the hours of 11 pm and 1 am. Also, your gallbladder dumps toxins during this same period. If you are awake, the toxins back up into your liver, which can further disrupt your sleep and your health.

• **Establish bedtime routine.** Could be meditation, prayer, deep breathing, aromatherapy, essential oils or a massage.

• **Best not to drink fluids 2 hours before bedtime.** This helps reduce frequency of needing to go to bathroom. Also make sure you **go to bathroom right before bed.** Elders – wise to have a handy pee-pot close to bed.

• **Have a high-protein soy drink several hours before bed.** This helps provide L-tryptophan needed for your melatonin and serotonin production (see page 182).

Is Electro-Magnetic Energy Hurting You?

A very wide array of symptoms have been attributed to EM exposure. Many complain of: Headaches, dizziness, memory loss, irritability, depression, anxiety, fatigue, muscle and joint pain, spasms, numbness, paralysis, strokes, insomnia, heart palpitations, irregular heartbeat, increased blood pressure, shortness of breath, sinus problems, asthma, bronchitis, shortness of breath, pain or burning of the eyes, blurred vision, cataracts, skin rash, burning, flushing itching, miscellaneous testicle or teeth pain, nosebleeds, hair loss, ringing in the ears, thyroid illness. It has been suggested, but not confirmed, that cell phones kept in pants are linked to testicular cancer and lower sperm counts. Try not to live or work close to high-tension electric wires, TV stations, or cell phone towers. The best thing to do if you are seriously ill is to check out other areas that do not cause symptoms. If some areas of your town are badly polluted with high-tension wires or other sources of EM Energy it is best to cut your losses and move to a place where you feel fine as soon as possible. Nothing is as important as retaining or regaining your health.

• **Avoid before bed: snacks, particularly grains and sugars.**

• **Take a hot bath, shower or sauna before bed.** The temperature drop from getting out of the bath or shower helps to signal your body it's time for bed and sleep.

• **Wear socks to bed.** Study shows wearing socks reduces night wakings. You could put hot water in Bragg ACV Drink glass bottle at feet at night. It's so comforting – PB!

• **Put work away at least one hour before bed.** This gives your mind a chance to unwind so you can go to sleep feeling calm, not hyped up or anxious about tomorrow's deadlines.

• **No TV hour before bed.** TV disrupts pineal gland function.

• **Keep Daily Journal.** (See page 151) Write in morning when brain is functioning at its peak and cortisol levels are high.

Lifestyle Suggestions That Enhance Sleep

• Avoid stimulants: caffeine (in coffee, some teas, even green teas, soft drinks, chocolate, sugar) and nicotine (found in cigarettes and other tobacco products).

• Don't drink alcohol to "help" you sleep, it's unhealthy!

• Have herbal teas – anise, lemon balm, Sleepytime, chamomile (beware some Green Teas have caffeine), or try melatonin, tryptophan (5HTP), valerian, calcium and magnesium supplements; they work miracles.

• Exercise regularly, but try to be finished with your workout no sooner than 2 hours prior to bedtime.

• Avoid foods you may be sensitive to. Reactions can cause excess congestion, gastrointestinal upset, bloating or gas.

• Associate your bed with recharging sleep – it's best not to sit on it to work or watch TV. *Try a memory 2" foam topper (so comfortable) on your firm mattress.*

• If you suffer from insomnia, don't nap during the day. Remember, earn better sleep by exercise and day activity.

Knowing these teachings will mean true life and good health. – Proverbs 4:22

Humor and Laughter is healthy – improves blood circulation, boosts immune system, and helps relieve stress. – Dr. Joel Goodman, Author of "Laffirmations"

Nervous Tension can ruin your health in dozens of ways and diminish your productivity and even shorten lifespan. – Dr. E. Jacobson, "You Must Relax"

Get Peaceful Sleep – Stop Snoring

 If snoring is happening frequently it can affect the quantity and quality of your sleep and that of family members. Snoring can lead to poor sleep, daytime fatigue, irritability, and increased health problems.

Where Does Snoring Come From?

People who snore often have too much throat and nasal tissue, or "floppy" tissue that is more prone to vibrate. The position of your tongue can also get in the way of smooth breathing. Snoring happens when you can't move air freely through your nose and mouth during sleep. Often caused by narrowing of your airway, either from poor sleep posture or abnormalities of the soft tissues in your throat. A narrow airway gets in the way of smooth breathing and creates the sound of snoring.

Common Causes of Snoring

Not all snoring is the same. Everyone snores for different reasons. When you understand why you snore, then you can better find the right solutions to a quieter sleep.

Age. As you reach middle age, your throat becomes narrower, and the muscle tone in your throat decreases.

The way you're built. Men have narrower air passages than women and are more likely to snore! A narrow throat, cleft palate, enlarged adenoids, obesity and other physical attributes contribute to snoring are often hereditary.

Nasal and sinus problems. Blocked airway passages with mucus, etc. can make breathing difficult and can create a vacuum in the throat, which can lead to snoring.

Being overweight or out of shape. Obesity, fatty tissue and poor body muscle tone can contribute to snoring.

Alcohol, smoking, and medications. Drinking alcohol, smoking, and certain medications can increase throat muscle relaxation which can lead to more snoring.

Sleep posture. Sleeping flat on back can cause flesh of throat to relax and block airway. Use head cradle pillow.

Is It Snoring or Is It Sleep Apnea?

Snoring could indicate sleep apnea, a potentially life-threatening condition that requires medical attention. Sleep apnea is a breathing obstruction, causing the sleeper to keep waking up to begin breathing again. Normal snoring doesn't interfere with the quality of your sleep as much as sleep apnea, so if you're suffering from extreme fatigue and sleepiness during the day, your problem may be more than just snoring, please seek medical advise (for more info on Sleep Apnea please read pages 102-104).

How You Snore Reveals Why You Snore

It's crucial to note different ways you sleep and snore! Sleep positions reveal a lot, and figuring out how you snore can reveal why you snore! Observing patterns in your snoring can often help pinpoint reasons why you snore, what makes it worse, and how to go about stopping your snoring.

• *Closed-mouth snoring* may indicate problem with tongue.

• *Open-mouth snoring* may be related to tissues in throat.

• *Snoring when sleeping on your back* is probably mild snoring. Start improving sleep habits and living The Bragg Healthy Lifestyle for the best and most effective cures.

• *Snoring in all sleep positions* can mean snoring is more severe and may require a more comprehensive treatment.

Some Self-Help Cures To Stop Snoring

There are many things you can do on your own to help you stop snoring. Home remedies and lifestyle changes can go a long way in resolving snoring health problems.

Lose weight. Losing even a little bit of weight can reduce the fatty tissue in the back of the throat and can help decrease or even stop your snoring.

Exercise can also help. Working out to tone your arms, legs, and abs, for example, also leads to toning the muscles in your throat, which in turn can lead to less snoring.

Quit smoking. If you smoke, chances of snoring and cancer are high. Smoking causes airways to be blocked by irritating membranes in the throat, sinus and nose.

Avoid alcohol, sleeping pills, and sedatives, especially before bedtime, because they relax the muscles in the throat and interfere with breathing. Talk to your doctor about any medications you're taking, as some encourage a deeper level of sleep which can make snoring worse.

Bedtime Remedies To Help You Stop Snoring

Clear nasal passages. Having a stuffy nose makes inhalation difficult and creates a vacuum in your throat, which can lead to snoring. Clear passages naturally with a Neti pot, ACV nasal wash or try nasal strips to help you breathe more easily while sleeping (pages 37-38).

Keep bedroom air moist with a humidifier. Dry air can irritate membranes in the nose and throat.

Reposition your neck. Elevating your head four inches may ease breathing and encourage your tongue and jaw to move forward. There are specially designed cradle pillows to help prevent snoring by making sure your neck and throat muscles are not crimped.

Memory Foam Pillows – available amazon.com

Avoid caffeine, heavy meals and drinking within 2 hours of going to bed, especially dairy products.

Sleep on side. Avoid sleeping flat on back, as gravity makes it more likely for your tongue and soft tissues to drop and obstruct your airway. *HelpGuide.org/life/snoring.htm*

A Different Kind of Relief for Snorer in the House

Now there are choices in treatments for relieving stubborn snoring. A simple doctor laser treatment could be the answer, or try – RIPSNORE™. A simple, one-piece device that molds to shape of mouth. The device is very flexible when being fitted. It stops snoring or drastically reduces snoring in 98% of people who started using it. The RIPSNORE™ holds lower jaw slightly forward, moving base of tongue away from back of airway and soft palate – allowing throat to be opened and snore to be silenced. The device is almost identical to dental ones, but is obviously a lot more affordable. See to order on web: *www.ripsnore.com.*

Somnoplasty: An Effective Treatment For Blocked Nasal Airways, Snoring & Sleep Apnea

Somnoplasty is a minimally invasive procedure that can be performed as an in-office surgery. It is done under local anesthesia with typical time lasting 15-20 minutes. The procedure involves using radio frequency heat to shrink relevant tissues leading to the shrinkage of inner tissues. For chronic nasal obstruction – the turbinates are targeted; habitual snoring the soft palate and uvula; and sleep apnea the base of the tongue and other airway structures. For more info: *Entsoa.com/Static/Somnoplasty_FAQ.html*

What Is Sleep Apnea?

Sleep apnea is a sleep disorder in which you have pauses in breathing or shallow breaths while you sleep. Breathing pauses can last from a few seconds to minutes. They often occur 5-30 times or more an hour. Typically, normal breathing then starts again. When you stop breathing, the balance of oxygen and carbon dioxide in the blood is upset. This imbalance stimulates the brain to restart the breathing process. The brain signals you to wake up so that the muscles of the tongue and throat can increase the size of the airway. Then, carbon dioxide can escape and oxygen can enter the airway. These waking episodes are necessary to restart breathing (and to save your life) and you my not remember them, but they do disrupt sleep and can cause daytime exhaustion.

Effects of Sleep Apnea on Your Health

Sleep apnea has serious health consequences and can be life-threatening. Please seek medical advise if you think you have sleep apnea. The main effects of sleep apnea are sleep and oxygen deprivation. With your breathing spurts your brain does not get enough oxygen. Problems can result from not getting enough oxygen, including: slow reflexes, poor concentration, and an increased risk of accidents. Also, heart disease, high blood pressure, stroke, diabetes, sexual dysfunction, weight gain and learning and memory problems (see box on page 96).

Sleep Apnea Signs and Symptoms

It can be tough to identify sleep apnea on your own, since most prominent symptoms only occur when you're asleep (you can try recording yourself during sleep). But some of the major signs and symptoms of sleep apnea are:

Pauses that occur while you snore, and if choking or gasping follows the pauses, these are major signs that you have sleep apnea! These breathing pauses typically last between 10-20 seconds and can occur up to hundreds of times a night, jolting you out of your natural sleep rhythm.

Another common sleep apnea sign is fighting sleepiness during the day, at work, or while driving. You may find yourself rapidly falling asleep during the quiet moments of the day when you're not active. Other common signs and symptoms of sleep apnea are:

• *Morning headaches*

• *Memory, learning and concentration problems*

• *Feeling irritable, depressed, or having mood swings*

• *Waking up frequently at night to urinate*

• *Dry mouth or sore throat when you wake up*

Some of the Risk Factors For Sleep Apnea

You have a higher risk for sleep apnea if you are:
- Overweight
- Male
- A smoker
- Hispanic, Black, or a Pacific Islander
- Related to someone who has sleep apnea
- Over the age of 65

Other risk factors include certain physical attributes, such as having a thick neck, deviated septum, receding chin, or enlarged tonsils or adenoids (the most common cause of sleep apnea in children). Your airway may be blocked or narrowed during sleep simply because your throat muscles tend to relax more than normal. Allergies or other medical conditions that cause nasal congestion and blockage can also contribute to sleep apnea.

Info from web: *HelpGuide.org/life/sleep_apnea.htm*

Help me to know the magic of rest and relaxation and restoring power of sleep.
– From poem "Slow Me Down, Lord" – Hittite prayer dating back 2000 years

Self-Help Treatment for Sleep Apnea

While a diagnosis of sleep apnea can be scary, it is a treatable condition! Minor sleep apnea is responsive to most self-health remedies, especially a healthy lifestyle. Some of the following treatments for sleep apnea might work for you:

1. **Lose Weight:** by losing even 10%, you can often help reduce sleep apnea and improve your sleep quality.

2. **Stop using alcohol, tobacco and sedatives:** these relax the muscles of the throat, also encouraging snoring.

3. **Sleep on your side:** those who have apnea usually experience sleep apnea when they sleep flat on back.

4. **Elevate the head of your bed 4 to 6 inches:** This can help alleviate snoring and make breathing easier.

5. **Maintain regular sleep hours.** Sticking to a steady sleep schedule will help you relax and sleep better. Apnea episodes decrease when you get plenty of sleep.

6. **Use nasal dilator, *BreatheRight.com* strips or make saline or ACV Nasal Wash** (page 37) or use Neti Pot or NeilMed (see *NeilMed.com*) squeeze bottle to help keep nasal passages open.

Healthy Mind Habit:

Wake up and say – Today I am going to be happier, healthier and wiser in my daily living! I am the captain of my life and am going to steer it to living a 100% healthy lifestyle! Fact is happy people look younger & have fewer health problems! – Patricia Bragg, ND, PhD., Pioneer Health Crusader

Slow, deep breathing and relaxation techniques are important health benefits to the entire body's system. Such techniques as sitting quietly, ignoring distracting thoughts, meditating and praying can bring down blood pressure and these healthy habits have no side effects. – Harvard Health Letter

Lavender helps you relax! *Before drying off after night bath or shower, place 3 drops of lavender essential oil on damp washcloth and rub it gently over body. The soothing active agents in lavender oil will enter body through skin and nose.*

The Serenity Prayer

God, grant me the serenity to accept
  the things I cannot change,
The courage to change the things I can,
And the wisdom to know the difference. – *Reinhold Niebuhr*

Chapter 15

Unhealthy Buildings and Homes Cause Many Breathing and Health Problems

Because we human beings have managed to pollute the water, air, and earth, our Mother Nature suffers! We know now that to stay healthy we must take precautions in some areas when we go in the great outdoors – or even in our backyard! But, it is probably a surprise to most people that even the "great indoors" can be unhealthy and polluted also! Studies show many homes and buildings are so toxic they are unfit to live in and work in.

Today unfortunately many modern homes, buildings, and even new cars (see page 107) that protect us from elements contain invisible toxic vapors that cause health problems as they give shelter! Contamination sources are many – and sadly often far too unrecognized and unaddressed!

Beware of Toxic Building Materials

Toxic building materials are the major source of environmental contaminants inside our homes, schools and places of business! For years unknowing builders have used many dangerous substances! Building materials, such as particle board, asbestos, and treated wood, can pose serious health threats. Other deadly substances include **roofing materials** and **insulation** – especially those made with **formaldehyde**, because they leak poisonous vapors! In addition, the horrors of **lead paint** (*www2.epa.gov/lead*) still threaten many people living in older homes. Lead is a highly toxic metal that may cause a range of health problems, especially in young children! When lead is absorbed into the body, it can cause damage to the brain and other vital organs, like the kidneys, nerves and blood.

The preservation of health is a duty. Few seem conscious that there is such a thing as responsible physical morality. – Herbert Spencer

---

Pollutants may negatively react chemically with body's tissues. – Dr. Andrew Weil

Formaldehyde Gives Off Toxic Vapors

Above your head, under your feet, on and in your walls, all around you in your home, formaldehyde could be poisoning your home and you. Formaldehyde is a colorless, strong-smelling gas. It is used to make building materials and household products. Formaldehyde is used to make walls, cabinets and furniture. Many contractors continue to use this toxic chemical as a preservative, binding agent and insulator. It turns up everywhere in our homes and buildings. Despite its widespread use, we know that formaldehyde is an eye, nose, throat and skin irritant – and is a strong suspected carcinogen! Formaldehyde can make you sick if you breathe it in too much. Symptoms can include: sore throat, cough, scratchy eyes and nosebleeds. Other symptoms include upper respiratory illnesses and allergies. **Formaldehyde is known to cause cancer.** Formaldehyde can irritate the airways, so people with asthma, bronchitis, or other breathing conditions are especially sensitive to toxic formaldehyde. (See web: *Cancer.gov/CancerTopics/FactSheet/Risk/Formaldehyde*

How do you cure your house of formaldehyde sickness? Unfortunately little can be done unless you build your house from scratch with careful attention to using only safe, natural building materials! Beyond this, only time will purify and heal the sick home. Over many years the toxic residues in building materials emit less harmful vapors, making older homes a healthier home – and the people who live there become healthier too. Our Santa Barbara home is over 100 years old.

Beware of Invisible Radon Gas Dangers

Like formaldehyde, radon is an invisible killer lurking in many homes, buildings and soil. Radon is a cancer-causing radioactive gas. You cannot see, smell or taste radon, but it may be a problem in your home. The Surgeon General has warned that radon is the second leading cause of lung cancer in the United States today. If you smoke and your home has high radon levels, you're at high risk for developing lung cancer! Also all natural stones and bricks used in construction should be checked for radon.

Although not much can be done, it's important to find out if your home has radon contamination! Contact local health department and ask if you live in high radon area. If you have concerns, ask to have a radon test done in home and surrounding area. Also ask about remedial actions. If home has high radon levels, seriously consider moving to a healthy home (friend got radon sickness and moved). Radon is second leading cause of lung cancer after smoking.

Check these websites for radon info: *www.radon.com* or *www.epa.gov/radon/pubs/citguide.html.*
These sites will take you to links on radon dangers.

Beware of Toxic Dangerous VOCs "Off-Gassing"

Off-gassing is the evaporation of toxic chemicals from: furniture, plastics, vinyl products, paints, office printers, cleaners and soaps, new car vapors, new clothing, cosmetics, mattresses, carpets, plywood and more.
Off-gassing emits Volatile Organic Compounds (VOCs), silent poison gasses and small particulate substances often throughout life of material. (web: *EcologyCenter.org*)

What about **synthetic carpets**? That soft carpeting that feels cozy to your feet is constantly shedding toxic vapors into your home. Carpets can emit VOCs for five years or possibly more, although the off-gassing decreases significantly several months after installation. The Environmental Protection Agency advises ventilating well for at least 72 hours after installation by opening windows and using fans that move air directly to the outdoors. Crawling toddlers are the most vulnerable!

Do not underestimate the dangers posed by **synthetic carpeting**! A young Honolulu attorney we knew was slowly paralyzed as a result of the **toxic vapors** given off from his new office carpeting. After several years of litigation, his wife and children finally won a large lawsuit against those responsible for his suffering and death.

The U.S. Environmental Protection Agency (EPA) and Surgeon General's Office have estimated that as many as 20,000 lung cancer deaths are caused each year by radon. Radon-induced lung cancer costs United States over $2 billion dollars per year in both direct and indirect health care costs. – radon.com

Formaldehyde exposures in carpets are often unrecognized causes of asthma, hay fever, and recurrent infections such as flu, plus many other less-suspected behavior symptoms. Visit: DrRapp.com "32 Tips That Could Save Your Life"

Healthy Home Environment is Important Check for Lead, Radon and Formaldehyde

Who wants to be sick and live in a sick home? You make the effort to eat well, sleep well and get exercise, don't drop the ball when it comes to ensuring a healthy living environment! **Here's some playing-it-safe ideas:**

First, be sure you and your family are safe from the dangers of *radon.* **Second,** be safe from the dangers of *formaldehyde;* older homes usually have less. Radon contamination is often worse in older homes. **Third,** be safe from the dangers of *lead paint* which is greater in older homes. Test for all three when considering a home. **Have licensed home inspector check for all three toxins** and others that might be sickening home, building, or apt., etc. you will or might live in. **It's reasonable and important!**

Don't cover floors with *toxic carpeting.* If you must put something on wood floors, safest are carpets and area rugs made from natural materials, wool or cotton. Don't cook with gas in an *unventilated room.* Be sure that your gas flame burns a clean blue. If you cook in a closed room with an orange flame you and your house will suffer from carbon dioxide, carbon monoxide, and other toxins.

To make a safe, happy and healthy home, spend the money to equip your house with plenty of windows and doors! Remember what the good doctor said for centuries: *Plenty of clean, fresh air is one of the best cures!* Keep your house well ventilated so that there can never be a poisonous buildup of dangerous toxins! Because poisons are often carried around the home by dust particles, **it's wise to buy a home air purifier that removes these toxic particles.**

MORE ON LEAD PAINT: *Lead is a toxic metal that can cause serious health problems if ingested or if dust containing lead is inhaled. Lead has been used in a wide variety of products found in and around our homes, including paint, ceramics, pipes and plumbing materials, gasoline, batteries, ammunition, and cosmetics. Up until 1978, when federal regulations restricted the use of lead in household paint, lead was a common component in exterior and interior paints. Lead can affect almost every organ and system in your body. Even low levels of lead in the blood of children can result in: behavior and learning problems; lower IQ and hyperactivity; slowed growth; hearing problems; and anemia.*

Toxic Chemicals Found In Your Home

Many toxic chemicals from household products can be found right in your home. Products such as detergent, floor and furniture polish, paints, and various cleaning products for glass, wood, metal, ovens, toilets and drains often contain toxic chemicals and vapors. Air fresheners can contain chemicals harmful to your health. These chemicals may include: ammonia, sulfuric and phosphoric acids, lye, chlorine, formaldehyde, petroleum solvents, and chlorinated phenols! If you have children also consider their art supplies, such as markers, paint and glue. Home furnishings, such as carpets, curtains, wall decorations, and some furniture may be treated with chemicals that are potentially dangerous.
(see web: *www.CEHN.org/education/toxic_products*)

Cleaning Supplies Can Affect Your Health

Many cleaning supplies or household products can irritate the eyes, the throat, cause headaches and other health problems. Some products release dangerous chemicals or gasses (vapors), including volatile organic compounds (VOCs). Other harmful ingredients include ammonia and bleach. *CAUTION: Never mix bleach with ammonia – the gasses created from this combination can lead to death! Please read all labels – it could save your life!* Even natural fragrances such as citrus (bathroom sprays often have citrus) that can produce dangerous vapor pollutants in your home.

VOCs and other chemicals released when using cleaning supplies contribute to chronic respiratory problems, allergic reactions and headaches. Studies are underway to assess how these chemicals affect people who have asthma and other respiratory illnesses. However, past studies link exposure to chemicals from cleaning supplies to asthma and other respiratory illnesses!

Products containing toxic VOCs and other toxic substances can include: aerosol spray products, including health, beauty and cleaning products; air fresheners; chlorine bleach; detergent and dish-washing liquids; dry cleaning chemicals; rug and upholstery cleaners; furniture and floor polish; and oven cleaners (see web: *lung.org*).

Chemicals, Toxic Vapors and Your Health

Each of us reacts differently to the chemical stew we face on a daily basis, and recognizing such health effects may be difficult! Typical reactions to new carpet VOCs include headaches, nausea, dizziness, shortness of breath, and asthmatic reactions. Longer-term effects also possible (see bottom paragraph page 107). CHE (Collaborative on Health and Environment – see below) lists benzene as having a strong link to leukemia and lymphomas, while styrene is associated with cognitive impairment and hearing loss, among other conditions. (web: *EcologyCenter.org*)

Some rules for minimizing VOCs in your home: Buy used goods if possible, the VOCs associated with their production have diminished over time, especially with cars, mattresses and furniture. Choose options like low- or no-VOC paint, which is now widely available and fairly economical! Always stay away from polyvinyl chloride, which is commonly found in linoleum, upholstery, and shower curtains (web: *EcologyCenter.org*).

An amazing resource – ***Collaborative on Health and the Environment (CHE) Toxicant and Disease Database*** (*HealthAndEnvironment.org*) is a searchable online database that summarizes links between chemical contaminants and approximately 180 human diseases or conditions. The CHE points out that more than 80,000 chemicals have been developed, distributed, and discarded into the environment over the past 60 years. Most have not been tested for toxic effects in humans or animals, and some are common in air, water, food, homes, work places, and sadly the communities we live in (web: *EcologyCenter.org*).

Steps to Reduce Exposure of VOC's: *Increase ventilation when using products that emit VOCs. Make sure to use household products according to manufacturer's directions. Throw away unused or little-used containers safely. Buy in quantities that you will use soon. Keep out of reach of children and pets. Never mix household care products unless directed on label.* – www.epa.gov

---

There are millions of allergic people in the U.S. About half of them feel their symptoms are severe enough to warrant professional help. – Dr. William Stuart

---

Chemicals play major role in our lives. They are part of what we eat, where we work and how we live. Despite their prevalence in our lives, many chemicals are toxic. Toxic chemicals can be found in our soil, water, air, and bodies. Contaminations seriously effect health of humans, pets and wildlife everywhere. – www.CEHN.org

Buy Healthy & Safe Products For Your Home

By cleaning out the toxins in your home, just like cleaning out toxins in our bodies, we create a space where energy can flow more easily. Replace toxic products with new improved eco-friendly ones that really work! Some of the worst and most common toxic offenders to watch out for are:

Ammonia – in window and other cleaners. Ammonia can cause coughing, wheezing, nasal complaints, eye irritation, throat discomfort and skin problems. In study, mice suffered from swelling and bleeding in lungs after 6 weeks exposure. **Alternatives:** We use white vinegar.

Chlorine – in water, bleach and cleaners – attacks organic matter (you are organic), skin and mucous membrane irritant. **Alternatives:** In shower use chlorine-removing shower filter (page 141), and use hydrogen peroxide-based bleaches.

Formaldehyde – in new furniture and carpeting – human carcinogen, causes birth defects, asthma and headaches. **Alternatives:** Seek old beautiful furniture available at moving sales and thrift stores. Buy old oriental rugs on *ebay.com*. They last so much longer and save you money in long run.

Anti-bacterial soaps – used in bathrooms and at work – breeds stronger, more dangerous bacteria by only killing weaker bacteria. **Alternative:** Use Castile all-natural soaps.

Check these websites for natural, healthy, safe products:

✔ *RealGoods.com*   ✔ *GoodGuide.com*
✔ *Shaklee.com*   ✔ *EcoMall.com*
✔ *GreenHome.com*   ✔ *SeventhGeneration.com*
✔ *BuyGreen.com*   ✔ *EarthEasy.com*

Asthma Linked to Home Environment

Over 25 million Americans experience frightening attacks of wheezing and breathlessness that are sometimes fatal. Asthma is not just one disease. Sometimes it's from an allergy and sometimes it's food related. Study shows Asthma is tied to what's inside your home, toxic products, sprays, etc., your genes, childhood infections, diet, milk, sugars, fast foods, and even stress! See pages 85-89 for more information on asthma and how to treat it naturally for miracle healings!

Exposure to formaldehyde causes eye, nose, and throat irritation, asthma, coughing, skin rashes, headaches, dizziness, nausea, vomiting and nosebleeds. – DrRapp.com

Enjoy Having a Healthy, Safe Home and More

Ensuring that your home is a healthy and safe space for you and your family is not an easy task. But what job could be more rewarding than health, happiness, vitality and a long, productive life? Creating a healthy home might not be inexpensive. However the savings in health care costs, lost productivity, worry and stress will greatly outweigh the short-term costs of making your home a safe haven. **Your home should be your Shangri-la Health Retreat.**

After you've done what you can about toxic walls and vapors, carpets, appliances, etc., here's more suggestions to help reduce home's toxicity. Read labels of all cleaning products, sprays, etc. Most are full of toxic ingredients, this includes detergents, soaps, fabric softeners, polishes, upholstery, carpet, oven cleaners and air fresheners, etc. Using toxic household cleansers, fly, ant, bug and moth balls, etc. can expose people to harmful vapors! Beware of ammonia, turpentine, paint, acetone, chlorine, sodium hydroxide, bleach, gasoline and all toxic vapors. Toss or store toxic products in garage. If you need to use any of these substances, consider only safe, non-toxic, natural versions! (webs page 111)

Important To Use Safe Pest and Weed Control

Pesticides and weed control products used around the home can cause a vast array of health problems! If pesticide sprays are being applied in your area, do the following:

1. Go to another section of town for 24-48 hours.
2. Do not allow pets or children outside on the lawn for at least 24 hours after the spraying.
3. If you must stay home, close all doors and windows and turn off air conditioning. If sensitive, seal these.
4. Use a fan in bedroom (mosquitoes do not like a breeze).

Researchers are looking at many irritants – like latex, which sloughs off automobile tires as tiny particles that may end up in your lungs. Some city studies pinpointed cockroaches as key allergens. Energy conservation has locked us in sick, "tight" closed-up office buildings and homes with sick, stale air, environmental toxins, gas appliances, secondhand smoke, pet hair and dander, mites, mold, and bacteria-laden dust.

Two healthy substitutes to use for household cleansers, deodorizers and disinfectants are baking soda and white vinegar. For safe, non-toxic formulas, techniques and products for cleaning your home check this web: EarthEasy.com

Chapter 16

Air Pollution & Smog

The Urgent Problems of Air Pollution

These days it doesn't matter where in the world you live or where you go, you can no longer absolutely escape exposure to the poisons that we humans have mindlessly dumped into our air, water and land. In pristine Minnesota, your water might be dangerously contaminated from upstream paper pulp mills. On beautiful New Guinea beaches, you might have to step around hazardous garbage carried great distances by ocean tides. Toxic waste by-products from oil production are found everywhere in the Middle East Deserts.

What these places all have in common from India to Mexico, from California to London and China, is air pollution! This is the greatest toxic scourge of modern man. Some areas are far worse than others. My recent travels bring London and Los Angeles smog to mind. Smoke contamination of the early industrial revolution compared to today's more deadly toxic chemical revolution is almost out of control! When air pollution toxins can actually be seen, then it's called *smog*.

What Is Smog?

Smog is a general term that refers to the various kinds of visible air pollution! The word *smog* – a combination of the words *smoke* and *fog* – was first invented in Glasgow, Scotland in the early 1900's. It described the thick, bad air that plagued and continues to plague their city. This smog killed over 1,000 people in 1909! Smog today is more complex than simply smoke mixed with fog. Many of these toxic deadly pollutants are invisible to the eye. Reread pages 105-110. Visit *www.epa.gov* or *www.arb.ca.gov*

According to the EPA, cars and trucks contribute more than 50% of the locally-generated air pollution. The remainder comes from solvent evaporation, surface cleaning and coating, petroleum production and other mobile sources (boats, trains, planes), combustion engines and other miscellaneous sources.

Pure, clean air is invisible staff of life! Smog is invisible staff of death!

Ground-level Ozone is Deadly Health Hazard

Breathing smoggy air can be hazardous because smog contains ozone, a pollutant that can harm our health when there are elevated levels in the air we breathe. Ozone is a colorless gas composed of three atoms of oxygen. Ozone can be good or bad, depending on where it is found:

Good Ozone: occurs naturally in the Earth's upper atmosphere - 1 to 30 miles above the Earth's surface - where it forms a protective layer that guards plant and animal life from the sun's damaging ultraviolet radiation.

Bad Ozone: in the Earth's lower atmosphere, near ground level, ozone is formed when industrial pollutants emitted by cars, power plants, industrial boilers, refineries, chemical plants and other sources react with sunlight, a dangerous chemical reaction occurs! At ground-level, where we eat, breathe and live, ozone combined with pollutants is responsible for smog's trademark "haze". This has a smothering toxic effect on the city dweller on smoggy days causing choking, coughing and eye-burning. Bad high ozone concentrations are especially harmful to children, the elderly, those with respiratory illnesses and people who exercise outdoors, walking, jogging, etc. in smog.

Ground-level Ozone: key component of smog, damages human lungs and body, animals, crops, even buildings and paint. Scientists have been studying effects of ozone on human health for many years! (*epa.gov/GroundLevelOzone*) Studies show Ozone promotes dangerous health effects:

1. *Ozone can irritate the entire respiratory system.* You might start coughing and feel irritation in your throat, and experience an uncomfortable sensation in your chest.
2. *Ozone can reduce lung function.* It is more difficult for you to breathe as deeply and vigorously as you normally would.
3. *Ozone can aggravate asthma.* Ozone makes people more sensitive to allergens and reduces your lung function.
4. *Ozone can inflame and damage the lining of the lungs.*
5. *Ozone has many other effects on people's health,* such as chronic lung disease, emphysema and bronchitis. Ozone may reduce the immune system's ability to fight off bacterial infections in the entire respiratory system.

Dirty Air Cost California $28 Billion Annually

Clean air is a delicate balance of Nitrogen (78%), Oxygen (20%), with small amounts of Argon (1%), Carbon Dioxide (.03%), and traces of Neon, Helium, Methane, Krypton, and Sulfur Dioxide. Gases such as carbon dioxide, methane and sulfur dioxide are normal components of clean air – it is when they reach much higher dangerous concentrations that it makes the air polluted and harmful to environment and human life!

Air pollution has become world's biggest health risk, linked to 7 million deaths across the globe, according to World Health Organization (WHO). Outdoor pollution (from traffic fumes and coal-burning) and indoor pollution (from wood and coal stoves), kills more people than smoking, road deaths and diabetes combined. In U.S., air pollution causes about 200,000 early deaths a year, with emissions from vehicle transport causing 53,000 and power generation 52,000, with California suffering the most air pollution compared to other states, having 21,000 deaths a year. Exposure to "dirty" air can cause premature death, hospitalizations and respiratory symptoms, chronic and acute bronchitis, asthma, limiting a person's normal daily activity and increasing childrens' school absences and lost workdays.

"Dirty" air is not only harmful for human life, it's harmful to U.S. environment. The harm done by sulphur dioxide alone to crops in U.S. is estimated at more than $500 million yearly plus damage done by countless poisons we pour into rivers and seas in terms of reduced fish catches is colossal! Mercury alone is considered responsible for annual $1 billion's-worth of damage worldwide.

Premature ageing is a highly toxic condition caused by shallow breathing, toxic air, nutritional deficiencies, negative thinking and an unhealthy lifestyle!

California plans to fight Carcinogens in the air. Among the chemicals cited were benzene, carbon tetrachloride, chloroform and vinyl chloride. Carcinogens are apparently released into the atmosphere from industries, and autos, especially diesel trucks. Regulations will be aimed at these sources.

Breathing pure, clean air deeply gives you more energy, go-power and sparkles up your life. – Dr. Patricia Bragg, Health Crusader, Lifestyle Educator

Smog Affects Humans, Plants, Animals, Buildings

Pollution not only affects humans by destroying their respiratory, cardiovascular and neurological systems; it also affects nature, plants, fruits, vegetables, rivers, ponds, forests, bees, animals, etc., on which we highly depend on for survival. Smog impacts environment by killing innumerable animal species and green life as these take time to adapt to breathing and surviving in such toxic environments. It's crucial to control pollution as nature, wildlife, bees and human life are precious gifts to all mankind. See web: *conserve-energy-future.com*

When components of smog – sulphur dioxide, nitrogen oxides and ammonia, end up in plants, surface water and soils, this has a number of toxic consequences:

• Availability of nutrients through soil is likely to decrease.

• When acidity is high then more metals will dissolve in water. This can cause surface water to become polluted, which has serious health effects on aquatic plants, fish and animals. Example: Mercury can be dispersed by transport through surface water, causing it to accumulate in fish. Read more: *www.lenntech.com*

• Smog can damage all plant life by inhibiting plants' natural ability to make and store food through photosynthesis. When this process is compromised, plant growth, reproduction and general health of the plant suffers! Smog can weaken plants that are already sensitive and make them more susceptible to infections, diseases, habitat stressers and pests! As a consequence, plants can dry out and become unable to contribute to the greater ecosystem that they belong to. Smog can deplete agricultural crops such as vegetables, soybeans, wheat, tomatoes, peanuts, and cotton, etc.

Air pollution may be even more dangerous than experts have suspected. A new study reveals how tiny particles penetrate buildings and people's airways more quickly and deeply than previously known! We suggest you follow Bragg Super Power Breathing Exercises (pages 71-81) so you can improve your breathing clean air to help offset damage from pollution and help improve health and energy. – web: breathing.com

---

Your health is your true wealth. – Paul C. Bragg, ND, PhD.

Polluted Air Becomes Polluted Water

Ammonia gas can contribute to *Eutrophication* – excessive growth of nutrients, from deposition or run-off, into natural waters, creeks, rivers, or lakes. *Eutrophication* causes a dense growth of plant life and death of animal life from lack of oxygen. Overgrowth of this choking algae vegetation or algal blooms disrupt normal functioning of the ecosystem, causing problems such as a lack of oxygen in the water, needed for fish and other aquatic life to survive! Water then becomes cloudy, colored a shade of green, yellow, or brown.

Smog Damages Buildings and Materials

The most visible characteristic of cities plagued with smog is the black and soot-covered windows, walls and other exposed surfaces! Yet, other damages can be seen. Sulfur dioxide corrodes metal and stone . . . damaging machinery and industrial instruments, as well as destroying buildings, statues, and monuments! Moreover, ground-level ozone has been found to bleach paints and coatings on buildings.

"CHEMTRAILS" – Toxic Heavy Metal Lead – Must Stop Being Sprayed into America's Skies

According to EPA, a grand total of 571 tons of lead are dumped each year into the air from aircraft alone! The fuel that powers most propeller type aircraft, when burned is called "avgas". Tests show that avgas contains the following: Lead 48 ppm; Bromine 42.6 ppm and Chlorine 605.2 ppm. Lead is a highly toxic heavy metal that causes bone diseases, brain damage and cancer (see more on lead bottom of page 108).

Avgas fuel is *emitting 86.4 kg of lead daily* into our air, and that lead falls onto our farming soils, forests, lakes, rivers, oceans, playgrounds, etc. Avgas emissions are number one source of lead emissions into the skies of America. Let's work together to clean up our skies. Please protest the use of this toxic aviation fuel! see *NatrualNews.com*

Airplanes are spraying chemicals across our skies that are on OSHA hazardous list. CHEMTRAILS show positive for toxic aluminum, barium, bacteria, virus, molds, causing health problems! **Check web:** ChemTrails911.com

Top 24 Worst U.S. Cities for Ozone-Smog*

Los Angeles, Bakersfield, Fresno and Houston have the dirtiest air in the country, depending on the type of pollution measured, but cities across the country don't escape bad grades from the association's national air quality report card:

Rank	Metropolitan Area	Rank	Metropolitan Area
1	Los Angeles/Long Beach, CA	13	St. Louis, MO/Farmington, IL
2	Visalia/Porterville, CA	14	Tulsa/Bartlesville, OK
3	Bakersfield, CA	15	Cincinnati, OH/Wilmington, KY
4	Fresno/Madera, CA	16	Philadelphia, PA/Reading, NJ
5	Sacramento/Roseville, CA	17	El Centro, CA
6	Houston, TX	18	Louisville, KY/Madison, IN
7	Modesto/Merced, CA	19	Oklahoma City/Shawnee, OK
8	Dallas/Fort Worth, TX	20	Chicago/Naperville, IL
9	Washington, DC/Baltimore, MD	21	Pittsburgh/New Castle, PA
10	Las Vegas, NV/Henderson, AZ	22	Fort Collins, CO
11	Phoenix/Mesa/Scottsdale, AZ	23	Birmingham/Hoover, AL
12	New York NY/Newark NJ	24	Cleveland/Akron, OH

*Ranking Smog-Ozone Pollution based on information from: American Lung Associations - 2015 • *www.StateOfTheAir.org*

Do Know Air Quality Level in Your Area

Air quality is measured by a nationwide monitoring system that records concentrations of ozone and other pollutants. EPA "translates" the pollutant concentrations to a standard Air Quality Index (AQI). The higher the AQI value, the greater the danger! You may see the local AQI for ozone-smog reported in the weather section of local newspaper, television, radio station, or check website: *www.AirNow.gov.* Also if you have pollen allergies go to *Pollen.com* and enter your zip code to receive a 4-day allergen forecast for your area.

The Air Quaility Index (AQI)

Ozone Concentration	AQI Values	Air Quality Description
0.0 to 0.064	0 to 50	Good
0.065 to 0.084	51 to 100	Moderate
0.085 to 0.104	101 to 150	Unhealthy for Sensitive Groups
0.105 to 0.124	151 to 200	Unhealthy

Average adult breathes over 3,000 gallons of air daily. – epa.gov/air

Healthful Solutions to Air Pollution

How can you supply your lungs, blood and whole body with clean healthy oxygen in this modern era of air pollution? **Oxygen, our invisible staff of life, is the greatest purifier and detoxifier, and is the body's basic life force.** First you must protect and strengthen your nose, sinuses, and your lungs, first line of defense. Don't drink or eat any dairy products, for they increase mucus production and cause airway passages to swell! These conditions hinder your nose's ability to filter the air you breathe, which is needed to protect your lungs and health. Take care of your nose, sinuses and health! Also develop powerful lungs that can withstand the challenges of polluted air when you're in it.

Action 1 Do your Super Power Breathing Exercises in the early morning when air is cleaner and less contaminated.

Action 2 Regularly check air pollution levels in your area and plan accordingly. If you know "Air Quality Index" (see chart page 118) is going to be high, limit outdoor exercise.

Action 3 Avoid highly polluted areas during heavy smog.

Action 4 If you live in smoggy area (*moving is best when possible*), **it's important to install the best HEPA air filters available** – particularly in rooms you sleep, exercise and work in, office, etc; even have one in your car. Learn how to clean the filters and replace the pads so that they are always clean, washed and able to cleanse and purify the air. Move your room air purifier from room-to-room every six hours so the air in the entire house is cleaner.

Action 5 Keep indoor air clean as possible! Don't smoke or be around any smokers! Keep house free of smoke, dust, and mold. Make sure fumes from gas stoves and heaters are properly vented! Reduce use of chemical cleaners, insecticides, solvents and toxic paints.

Clean Air in Home, Office & Car. Many people are unaware that exposure to indoor pollutants at home, office, work & even new car vapors are often greater than levels found outdoors, causing serious health problems! Having air purifier helps eliminate bacteria, viruses, mold, & other indoor pollutants. Read "Consumer Reports" & visit webs for more info on clean home air: Oreck.com & IQair.com

---

Human beings breathe in and out about once every 4 seconds, 16 times a minute, 960 times an hour making up about 8.5 million times a year of air intake into their body. This adds air going into the body about 1 million gallons of oxygen-containing air every year from earth's surface.

Action 6 Keep yourself healthy. Stop smoking. Eat well and exercise regularly. Fortify yourself internally with a multiple vitamin-mineral supplement, ample vitamin C and especially vitamin E (natural d-alpha mixed tocopherols), the body's oxygen protector. One of the vital functions of vitamin E is to regulate the use of oxygen by the body's cells. This helps assure that your life-giving oxygen is properly utilized for essential energy and that a reserve is retained in the red corpuscles for use when extra effort is needed. According to documented medical research, vitamin E helps increase the energy potential of all the oxygen you breathe by an amazing 25% to 50%! (see pages 157-160)

Action 7 Best to live away and stay away from high traffic roads especially when on your daily brisk health walks.

Let's Clean-Up Our Air – For Our Health!

We can all help reduce ozone by taking the following steps:

- **Drive Less. Instead of a car, you may want to walk, use mass transit or ride a bike in safe bike lanes!**

- **Start a carpool want list and carpool when possible.**

- **Make sure your car is well-tuned**. Also take care not to over fill or spill gasoline when filling tank.

- **Make sure that you tightly seal** the lids of chemical products to keep the evaporation to a minimum.

Paving over land increases overall temperatures – and ozone forms more quickly at higher temperatures. More than one-half of commuting trips and 3 out of 4 shopping trips are less than 5 miles in length – perfect for cycling. For example: if Santa Barbara County could replace just 3% of its car and light truck trips with bike and walking trips, they could reduce emissions of smog-forming pollutants in this California County by 9 tons monthly.

Is there a relationship with breathing and diabetes, cancer, heart trouble, stress, asthma, emphysema, and other illnesses? YES! According to Framingham 30 year study that clarified breathing's direct relationship with longevity and fact that many will lose 75% of their breathing capacity by age 75, if they don't take action and learn easy and safe ways to breathe better (web: breathing.com).
It's best to follow our Super Power Breathing Exercises (pages 71-81).

We Need the Protection of the Clean Air Act!

In many ways the problem of smog is worse now than 50 years ago. Hopefully we will never have air pollution disasters on the scale of some in the past. No one wants to live through suffering like that of the disastrous London smog attack of December 1952. A thermal inversion settled a fog on this great city on the Thames, trapping the pollutants spewed from its heavy industries and thousands of chimneys. Before the crisis abated, more than 12,000 people were dead and countless had fallen ill. Hospitals were inundated with patients suffering from **Cyanosis, a condition in which a person actually turns blue for want of oxygen!**

Today we fortunately have national and local agencies whose job is to prevent such past horrible smog disasters! These agencies constantly monitor air pollutant levels and atmospheric conditions. Based on their findings, guidelines and legislation will be implemented to protect our health, but sadly problems do persist! Environmental Protection Agency (EPA) notes that a larger number of Americans are living in areas that don't meet air quality standards. Over 64 urban areas don't meet federal standards of air quality – standards which many say are not safe enough to keep our air healthy! (*www.epa.gov*)

Recently, EPA approved more protective air quality standards. Studies show back in 2010 Amendments of 1990 prevented 23,000 Americans from dying prematurely and averted over 1.7 million incidences of asthma attacks and aggravations of chronic asthma. In 2010 they prevented 67,000 incidences of chronic and acute bronchitis, 91,000 occurrences of shortness of breath, 4.1 million lost work days and 31 million days in which Americans would have had to restrict activity due to air pollution related illness! Because of 2014 new safer standards, many cities and urban areas will monitor air and become more alert to air pollution problems. It's best to become politically aware of all situations that affect your health in the area where you live! Vote for the laws and strong regulations that protect your health rights, especially to breathe clean, non-toxic air!

The clean energy laws will generate new jobs and save consumers money. California saved consumers $56 billion on household energy costs. With the smart energy policies that promote a transition to renewable energy sources such as wind and sun, California residents will benefit even more.

Clean Air Act Benefits and Costs

According to EPA's best 2020 estimate the *benefits* of Clean Air Act programs will total about $2 trillion. Benefits were looked at for a number of factors including – improved public health, avoided food crop damage, control of cancer-causing toxic air, the value of avoiding increases in illness and premature death, and the benefits to the ecosystem. The *cost* of achieving these health-saving and ecological benefits are likely to be about $1,886 billion. If the Clean Air Act Amendments had not been enacted by 1990, 205,000 Americans would have died prematurely! Yes, millions more would have suffered from asthma and respiratory illnesses ranging from mild to severe!

Throughout the Clean Air Act, questions have been raised as to whether the health benefits of air pollution control justify the costs incurred by industry and taxpayers. The broader question is simple: How do the overall health, welfare, ecological and economic benefits of the *life-saving* Clean Air Act compare to these high cost programs? **The saving of human and animal health and food crops is reason enough to continue with programs to clean up the air we breathe and to protect lives and food crops!**

The results indicate that the benefits of the Clean Air Act and associated control programs substantially exceeded costs ($114 billion). A second important implication of this study is that a large proportion of the cost benefits of the Clean Air Act reducing comes in two major smog pollutants: lead and particulate matter. Not only monetarily, but from a health standpoint as well, **the Clean Air Act is vitally needed and important to our health and well-being!!!**

Negative factors like air smog, soil and water pollutants, acid rain, UV radiation caused by the depletion of the earth's protective ozone layer, chemically treated foods, the disturbance of immune systems through repeated toxic vaccination and immunization, not to mention our stress-infused lifestyles, result in reduced immune response and the inability of our bodies to cope with or neutralize allergens. – Dr. Linda Page – *Allergy Control & Management*

We all grow healthier in nature, healthy foods, pure air, gentle sunshine and love!

My love of nature's beauty blesses me and gives me strength. – Paul Bragg, ND, PhD.

Chapter 17

Doctor Natural Foods
Eating for Super Health, Energy and Longevity

Natural nutrition and correct breathing habits together will lift you to higher levels of health vibration for happy, healthful living! To attain and maintain the peak of Super Health, we practice and recommend eating two balanced, healthy meals per day and taking a 24 to 32 hour distilled water cleansing fast each week. (Read pages 144, 147.)

Upon arising, before doing our Super Power Breathing Exercises, we drink the Bragg Apple Cider Vinegar Drink: 2 tsps of ACV and raw honey (optional) in a glass of distilled water (page 149). Read Bragg *Apple Cider Vinegar* book for more info on the miracle uses – page 34, 237-239.

After our breathing exercises we try to get from one to three hours of outdoor exercise: brisk walking, biking, swimming, hiking, weightlifting, gardening. Then we have fresh fruit or the Bragg Energy Pep Drink (page 149) before we get busy; writing, doing radio talk shows by phone, etc.

Our first real meal comes about mid-day. This gives the stomach a thorough rest of 16 to 18 hours, allowing it time to completely empty, recuperate and accumulate an abundant supply of new digestive juices after previous evening's meal. Relax and chew each mouthful of food thoroughly *(remember stomach has no teeth)* so the digestive process will have a good start, so your food will be well assimilated to give you the health and energy needed!

Let food be your medicine and medicine be your food. Nature heals; the physician is only nature's assistant. – Hippocrates, 400 BC

Excess body fat is linked to killer diseases – such as high blood pressure, diabetes, stroke and heart attack. Apple Cider Vinegar (ACV) also contains natural occurring acetic acid, the primary ingredient in vinegar. Studies show (ACV) boosts metabolism and helps dissolve body fat (pg. 240).

Enjoy healthy, organic foods for their wonderful abundance of life energy.

Now learn what great benefits a temperate diet will bring with it. In the first place, you will enjoy good health. – Horace, 65 B.C.

The journey of a thousand miles begins with one step. – Lao Tzu

Power Salad for Lunch – Gives Energy & Health

A healthy, large salad of raw fruits or raw garden vegetables (organically grown is best) with raw nuts, sunflower or sesame seeds, soy or feta goats cheese for protein is an ideal delicious luncheon. Try our favorite Bragg Salad and Salad Dressing Recipes on page 150.

Most Americans have schedules which don't permit resting after midday meal. But in Spain, Mexico and many countries worldwide, the main meal is at midday and is followed by a siesta. This short nap is ideal, giving you almost two fresh days in one! Rushed Americans eat their main meal in the evening and sadly millions eat a quick, unhealthy meal at fast food restaurants at noon.

Enjoy Healthy, Balanced Variety for Dinner

Relax at day's end with some Super Power Breaths. Cleanse the toxins from your lungs so that you will get the full benefit from a well-balanced, healthy nourishing and tasty dinner! Your basic health menu should include:

Salad: A smaller serving this time of fresh raw vegetables and salad greens or try one of these suggestions:
- Sliced red and green cabbage with diced red and green bell peppers and grated carrots
- grated carrots, sliced raw apples and raisins or try grated carrots, raisins, and diced pineapple
- lettuce, tomato, avocado and cucumber salad

Prepare Bragg Salad Dressing Recipes or try New Bragg Organic Ginger & Vinaigrette Dressings – page 242. Sometimes we just squeeze orange or lemon over salads and spray Bragg Aminos and Nutritional Yeast over top – delicious!

Cooked Vegetables: Include green and yellow veggies; lightly cook, steam, bake, wok or stir-fry. Season with Bragg Liquid Aminos and Salad Dressings (page 242), Bragg Sprinkle (24 herbs & spices) or Bragg Kelp, for taste delights.

Protein Dish: Vegetable proteins include all beans, brown rice, lentils, tofu, etc., and raw, unsalted nuts and seeds. We recommend a vegetarian diet. If you do eat meat, limit it to 3 times a week and start becoming a vegetarian.

America badly needs to go on a healthy diet. We should do something about excessive, life-threatening fat. We should get rid of harmful obesity in quickest possible way and this is by fasting (page 147). – Allan Cott, M.D.

Healthy Plant-Based Daily Food Guide

Be a Bragg Crusader – copy and share with friends, clubs, etc.

- **CALCIUM - RICH FOODS**
  4-6 Servings

- **VEGETABLES**
  2/3 raw 1/3 cooked
  6-8 Servings

- **WHOLE GRAINS, CEREALS, PASTA & BROWN RICE**
  1-3 Servings

- **OMEGA - 3 FATTY ACIDS**
  FLAXSEEDS
  VITAMIN D3
  VITAMIN B12

- **BEANS, LEGUMES NUTS & SEEDS & ALTERNATIVES**
  2-3 Servings

- **FRUITS**
  (especially Apples & the skin)
  4-6 Servings

- **WATER**
  8 Glasses

8 Glasses Daily Purified/Distilled Water

Never add table salt! Prepare your foods with healthy, nutritious flavors from fresh garlic, onions, herbs and Bragg Sprinkle (24 herbs & spices), Bragg Kelp and Bragg Liquid Aminos made from healthy non-GMO soy beans.

Dessert: If desired, fresh organic fruits (apples, pears, etc.) are best when available, or unsweetened, stewed or dried fruit. For special desserts make one of the healthy pies, cakes, cookies, etc., in our *Bragg Vegetarian Health (700) Recipe Book*.

Beverages: For health, it's best not to drink beverages with meals, not even water! Your digestive juices do their best work undiluted! Have ample fluids hour before and hour after meals and during daytime. At least an hour after dinner, you may have the delicious Bragg Apple Cider Drink (hot or cold), herbal tea or a glass of fresh fruit or vegetable juice, if you wish. Drink all the distilled water you want between meals – ideal is 8 glasses daily!

Paul Bragg Talks about Vinegar Miracles on Large Family Farm in Youth.
Long years of research have proven to me that natural apple cider vinegar is a good source of potassium. I was raised on a large farm where we grew many varieties of delicious apples we all enjoyed. Each year my father made natural apple cider vinegar and stored it in wooden barrels. On our table we used this natural apple cider vinegar on foods and enjoyed daily vinegar drinks and our family thrived and loved it.

Eating Apples Can Give You Burst of Energy. *Researchers found significant boost in endurance capacity from quercetin in red apples. Quercetin (a phytonutrient see page 130) is a natural antioxidant that boosts the power of the mitochondria (the powerhouse of the cell) in muscles and the brain. This surge of power gives you energy!*

125

Start Eating Healthy Foods For Super Energy

The *Healthy Plant-Based Daily Food Guide Pyramid* illustration (previous page) represents an ideal way of eating for achieving optimal nutrition, health and longevity! You will notice that this Food Guide Pyramid is based on healthy organic plant-based foods, with the emphasis on purified water, fruits, vegetables, whole grains, vegetable protein foods, non-dairy calcium foods, and raw nuts and seeds. This is best diet for heart wellness, disease prevention and to enjoy longevity. *Eating a diet based on these dietary guidelines will help you get the nutrients needed for optimal health!*

• **Purified/Distilled Water:** Is pyramid's foundation. We recommend *distilled water,* as it's the purest water for the body! Drink eight – 8 oz glasses of distilled water daily and even more if your lifestyle (sports, work, etc.) requires it.

• **Whole Grains:** Whole grains are pyramid's next level. Avoid all process, refined GMO grain products and eat only unrefined, organic whole grain bread and cereal products! Grains such as quinoa, whole wheat, brown rice, barley, oats, millet, kamut, as well as 100% whole grain breads and cereals are best. One serving of whole grains is equal to 1 slice whole grain bread, 1 ounce ready-to-eat whole grain cereal, 1 cup cooked whole grains such as brown rice, oatmeal or other grains, 1 cup 100% whole wheat (or other whole grains) pasta or noodles, and 1 ounce of other whole grain products. We recommend eating 1-3 servings of organic, non-GMO whole grains daily.

• **Vegetables:** We recommend eating as many of your vegetables organic and raw (uncooked, in salads, juices, smoothies, etc.) as possible! When cooking vegetables, don't overcook them! Steaming or lightly stir-frying is best. The more colorful rainbow of vegetables you eat is better for your health as they contain more valuable healthful phytonutrients (see page 130). Eat a wide variety of organic vegetables daily. One vegetable serving is equal to 1 cup cooked vegetables or 1 cup raw uncooked vegetables, 1 cup salad, or 3/4 cup vegetable juice. We recommend having 6-8 or more vegetable servings daily.

The secret of longevity is eating intelligently healthy. – Gaylord Hauser

●**Fruits:** Like vegetables, the more colorful the fruits the better they are for you. Enjoy organic fruits as much as possible! One serving of fruit is equal to 1 medium apple, banana, orange, pear or other fruit, $1/2$ cup fruit, $1/2$ cup of fruit juice or $1/4$ cup dried fruit. We recommend eating 4-6 servings or more of organic fruits daily.

●**Calcium-Rich Foods:** Are plant-derived calcium-rich foods. Plant sources of calcium are healthier than dairy products because they don't contain saturated fats or cholesterol. Health calcium-rich foods are: soymilk, tofu, broccoli and green leafy vegetables. Examples of serving sizes of plant-derived calcium-rich foods include: 1 cup soymilk, $1/2$ cup tofu, $1/3$ cup almonds, 1 cup cooked or 2 cups high calcium dark greens (kale, collards, broccoli, bok choy or other Chinese greens), 1 cup calcium-rich beans (soy, white, navy, Great Northern), $1/2$ cup seaweed, 1 tablespoon blackstrap molasses, 5 or more figs. We recommend having 4-6 servings of healthy non-dairy sources of calcium rich foods daily.

●**Beans, Legumes, Nuts & Seeds:** This group are the healthy protein foods. Vegetable protein foods are more optimal compared to animal protein foods. Vegetable proteins do not contain the artery clogging saturated fats and cholesterol found in animal foods. They also contain protective factors to help prevent heart disease, cancer and diabetes. Vegetable proteins are high quality and provide the body with the essential amino acids that it requires. One serving of vegetable protein foods include: 1 cup cooked legumes (beans, lentils, dried peas), $1/2$ cup firm tofu or tempeh, 1 serving of "veggie meat" alternate (e.g. veggie burger patty or soy patty), 3 tablespoons nut or seed butter, 1 cup soy milk. We recommend you have 2 to 3 or more vegetable protein servings daily with meals.

Life cannot be maintained unless life be taken in. And this is best done by making at least 60% of your diet raw and with a plentiful supply of fresh juicy organic fruits and some lightly cooked vegetables. – Patricia Bragg, ND, PhD.

Grains that are heart-healthy are organic brown rice, organic whole grain breads, cereals, and pastas. There's also buckwheat, barley, millet, and tasty quinoa is a complete protein and makes an ideal breakfast cereal. Also popcorn, organic corn is a whole grain. My favorite is air-popped and top with Bragg Liquid Aminos, Olive Oil and Nutritional Yeast (recipe page 149).

Bragg Healthy Lifestyle helps make a healthier you and a healthier world!

•Healthy Fats, Essential Fatty Acids, Omega-3 and Other Nutrients: Servings of healthy fats include: 1 tsp flaxseed oil (flaxseed is high in phytonutrients called lignans), 1 Tbsp of Bragg Organic Extra-Virgin Olive Oil, 3 tsps raw walnuts. Other healthy essentials include nutritional B-Complex supplements that provide vitamin B12, that Bragg Nutritional Yeast has (delicious seasoning). Do provide your body with nutritional supplements your body requires for optimal health (see page 182).

What are Nature's Miracle Phytonutrients?

These wonderful, organic compounds are found in plants, ('phyto' means 'plant' in Greek), that are vital to human health. Increasingly, scientific studies are showing that phytonutrients help protect us from many serious health issues, including heart disease and stroke. Organic fruits, vegetables, grains, legumes, nuts, seeds and some teas are rich in the miracle phytonutrients.

Physicians and Scientists have written about the critical nature of these foods for thousands of years, but the specific benefits of phytonutrients are still being discovered. They are created when plants absorb energy from the earth, water, air and sun. This energy helps plants survive environmental challenges such as diseases, injures, drought, excessive heat, ultraviolet sunrays and poisons. This incredible energy forms an important part of the plant's immune system! It appears to provide humans with the same benefits, when we consume the plants! They help increase our immune and regeneration systems. **Plants give us strength, endurance, health and ultimately help us feel better and live longer.**

To Make Organic Nut Butters:

Grind 1 1/2 cups of raw unsalted organic nuts in a food processor or blender. Continue grinding nuts down until they are a thick, fudge-like paste. Then add sunflower or nut oil (start with 1 Tbsp and add more only if necessary), blend until smooth. Best kept refrigerated.

Chia Seeds: *Bragg promoted in 1940 – are rich in omega-3 fatty acids and antioxidants! Chia seeds provide fiber and calcium, phosphorus, magnesium, iron, niacin and zinc. They help slow down how fast our bodies convert carbohydrates into simple sugars, which may have great benefits for diabetics.*

Antioxidants & Phytonutrients Health Benefits

The body must have these phytonutrients and enzymes to break food down, kill viruses and bacteria and dissolve tumors! A diet of at least 50% raw, unprocessed foods is vital to make sure that we are getting enough enzymes and phytonutrients to optimize the body's processes.

Plants contain more than 10,000 phytonutrients, one reason 10-14 servings of fruits and veggies daily are recommended. Plants and vegetables contain different phytonutrients, having a variety in diet is important.

On average, plant foods have 64 times more antioxidants than animal foods, which is critical because when it comes to antioxidants, the more we eat, our heath benefits! **Eating a diet high in antioxidants is important because they reduce inflammation and free radicals in the body** and help protect against heart disease and cancer. See chart page 130 for health benefits of different plant sources. See: *hsph.Harvard.edu/NutritionSource/antioxidants*.

Main Sources of Miracle Phytonutrients

The following are high in phytonutrients: carrots and yellow vegetables (sweet potatoes and pumpkins), peaches, apricots, broccoli, leafy greens (kale, spinach, turnip greens), tomatoes, pink grapefruit, watermelon, guava, blackberries, walnuts, strawberries, cranberries, raspberries, blueberries, grape juice, and prunes, red cabbage, pineapple, oranges, plums, pinto beans, spinach, kiwi fruit and red peppers.

The more live, unprocessed foods we eat the more phytonutrients and enzymes we consume the healthier our diet. This natural food is full of energy we need to live longer, healthier lives! To boost your immune system and cell regeneration eat more phytonutrients, practice deep breathing exercises daily, get physical exercise, and make sure your diet is at least 50% raw, healthy, organic foods! That's The Bragg Healthy Lifestyle and when followed produces miracles.

Increasing intake of fruits and vegetables can help you prevent heart disease, cancer and other chronic diseases. Surveys show those who increased their daily fruit and vegetable intake improved their health, vitality and well-being.
– UC Berkeley Wellness Letter • www.BerkeleyWellness.com

Nature's Miracle Phytochemicals Help Prevent Cancer:

Make sure to get your daily dose of these naturally occurring, cancer-fighting super foods – phytonutrients that are abundant in apples, tomatoes, onions, garlic, beans, legumes, soybeans, cabbage, cauliflower, broccoli, citrus fruits, etc. The champions with the highest count of phytonutrients go to apples and tomatoes.

Class	Food Sources	Action
PHYTOESTROGEN ISOFLAVONES	Soy products, flaxseed, seeds & nuts, yams, alfalfa & red clover sprouts, licorice root (not candy)	Helps block some cancers, & aids in menopausal symptoms and helps improve the memory
PHYTOSTEROLS	Plant oils: corn, sesame, safflower; rice bran, wheat germ, peanuts	Blocks hormonal role in cancers, inhibits uptake of cholesterol from diet
LIGNANS	Flaxseeds, rye, lentils, soy mushrooms, barley	Helps prevent cancer, heart disease and stroke
SAPONINS	Yams, beets, beans, cabbage, nuts, soybeans	Helps prevent cancer cells from multiplying
TERPENES	Carrots, winter squash, sweet potatoes, yams, apples, cantaloupes	Antioxidants – protects DNA from free radical-induced damage
	Tomatoes & its sauces, tomato-based products	Helps block UVA & UVB and offers help to protect against cancers – breast, prostate, etc.
	Spinach, kale, beet & turnip greens, cabbage	Protects eyes from macular degeneration
	Red chile peppers	Keeps carcinogens from binding to DNA
QUERCETIN (& FLAVONOIDS)	Apples (especially the skins), red onions & green tea	Strong cancer fighter, protects heart & arteries. Reduces pain, allergy & asthma symptoms
	Citrus fruits (flavonoids)	Promotes protective enzymes
PHENOLS	Apples, fennel, parsley, carrots, alfalfa, cabbage	Helps prevent blood clotting & has some anticancer properties
	Cinnamon	Promotes healthy blood sugar and glucose metabolism
	Citrus fruits, broccoli, cabbage, cucumbers, green peppers, tomatoes	Antioxidants – flavonoids, block membrane receptor sites for certain hormones
	Apples, grape seeds	Strong antioxidants; fights germs & bacteria, strengthens immune system, veins & capillaries
	Grapes, especially skins	Antioxidant, antimutagen; promotes detoxification. Acts as carcinogen inhibitors
	Yellow & green squash	Antihepatoxic, antitumor
SULFUR COMPOUNDS	Onions & garlic, (fresh is always best) Red onions (our favorite) also contain Quercetin	Promotes liver enzymes, inhibits cholesterol synthesis, reduces triglycerides, lowers blood pressure, improves immune response, fights infections, germs & parasites

The Bragg Healthy Lifestyle Promotes Super Health and Super Energy!

When you eat according to The Bragg Healthy Lifestyle, 60% to 70% of your diet will consist of fresh, raw, live foods (organic is best): Raw veggies, salads, fresh fruits and juices, sprouts, raw seeds and nuts. Enjoy 100% whole grain breads (home-baked is best), whole grain pastas and cereals, organic brown rice, beans and legumes. You can make healthy and delicious combination salads, soups, casseroles, etc., and the nutritious blender drinks that all ages will love. These are the healthy, no cholesterol, low-sodium live foods which provide good body fuel for more increased health and vitality. **These wholesome foods make joyous, healthy, energized people!**

Following The Bragg Healthy Lifestyle, you will become revitalized and reborn into a fresh new life filled with joy, vitality, youthfulness and longevity! There are millions of healthy Bragg followers around the world who have proven to themselves that this Healthy Lifestyle works miracles when followed faithfully. **For more info on the lifestyle that keeps you ageless, read the book** *Bragg Healthy Lifestyle – Vital Living to 120!* (See back pages for Bragg book list info).

Dr. Koop & Patricia

Hawaii Health Conference

Bad Nutrition – #1 Cause of Sickness

"Diet-related diseases account for 68% of all deaths."
– Dr. C. Everett Koop

America's former Surgeon General and our friend, said this in his famous 1988 landmark report on nutrition and health in America. People don't die of infectious conditions as such, but of malnutrition that allows the germs to get a foothold in sickly bodies! Also, bad nutrition is usually the cause of non-infectious, fatal or degenerative conditions. When the body has its full nutrition quota of vitamin and minerals, including potassium, it's almost impossible for germs to get a foothold in a healthy, powerful bloodstream and tissues!

Former U.S. Surgeon General, Dr. C. Everett Koop said –
"Paul Bragg did more for the Health of America than any one person I know."

Eliminating Meat is Safer and Healthier

Play it safe, become a healthy vegetarian! They feed cattle antibiotics, growth hormones and dead, ground up carcasses of other feed lot animals who didn't make it to the slaughterhouse. See informative web: *www.EarthSave.org.*

Also, consider the fact that cattle, sheep, chickens, etc., are all vegetarians by nature! When you eat them, you are just eating polluted vegetables. Why not skip all the waste and toxins and just eat healthy, organic vegetables?

Meat is also a major source of cholesterol and uric acid, both harmful to your health! If you are going to include meat in your diet, it should not be eaten more than two times a week. In our opinion, fresh fish can be the least toxic of flesh proteins. But beware of fish from polluted waters, they can be contaminated with mercury, lead, cadmium, dangerous pesticides and many other toxic substances. If you are unable to test the waters from where your fish come, don't risk eating them. And avoid shellfish – shrimp, lobster and crayfish. They are garbage-eating bottom-feeders – the rats and flies of the water kingdom. They eat the rotting, decaying scum and refuse off the bottoms of the oceans, lakes and rivers. Next comes chicken and turkey, don't eat the skin, it's heavy in cholesterol. Third place goes to lamb and beef. More shocking facts follow. People should not eat pork or pork products of any kind. The pig is the only animal besides man that develops arteriosclerosis or hardening of the arteries. In fact, this animal is so loaded with cholesterol that in cold weather, unprotected pigs will become stiff, and some die. This animal is often infected with a dangerous parasite that cause trichinosis disease.

FLASH *–Scientists agree that bacon, sausage and other processed meats and red meats cause cancer. World Health Organization (see web: WHO.int) study suggests that an additional 3.5 oz. of red meat everyday raises risk of colorectal cancer by 17%; eating an additional 1.8 oz. of processed meat daily raises risk by 18%. About 34,000 cancer deaths a year worldwide are attributable to diets high in processed meats. Red meat includes beef, veal, pork, lamb, mutton and goat. Process meat includes hot dogs, ham, sausages, corned beef and jerky.*

 Evidence shows that eating a meat based diet is bad for the environment, aggravates global hunger, brutalizes animals and compromises your health.

Plant-Based Protein Chart

BEANS & LEGUMES

(1 cup cooked)	PROTEIN IN GRAMS
Soybeans	29
Lentils	18
Adzuki Beans	17
Cannellini	17
Navy Beans	16
Split Peas	16
Black Beans	15
Garbanzos (chick peas)	15
Kidney Beans	15
Great Northern Beans	15
Lima Beans	15
Black-eyed Peas	14
Pinto Beans	14
Mung Beans	14
Tofu (3 oz.)	7 to 12
Green Peas (whole)	9

RAW NUTS & SEEDS

(1/4 cup or 4 Tbsps)	PROTEIN IN GRAMS
Chia Seeds	12
Macadamia Nuts	11
Flax Seeds	8
Sunflower Seeds	8
Almonds	7
Pumpkin Seeds	7
Sesame Seeds	7
Walnuts	5
Brazil Nuts	5
Hazelnuts	5
Pine Nuts	4
Cashews	4

NUT BUTTERS

(2 Tbsps)	PROTEIN IN GRAMS
Peanut Butter	7 to 9
Almond Butter	5 to 8
Cashew Butter	4 to 5
Sesame - Tahini	6

VEGETABLES

(1 Serving or 1 cup)	PROTEIN IN GRAMS
Spirulina	8.6
Corn (1 cob)	5
Potato (with skin)	5
Mushrooms, Oyster	5
Artichoke (1 medium)	4
Collard Greens	4
Broccoli	4
Brussel Sprouts	4
Mushrooms, Shitake	3.5
Swiss Chard	3
Kale	2.5
Asparagus (5 spears)	2
String Beans	2
Beets	2
Peas	2
Sweet Potato	3
Summer Squash	2
Cabbage	2
Carrot	2
Cauliflower	2
Squash	2
Celery	1
Spinach	1
Bell Peppers	1
Cucumber	1
Eggplant	1
Leeks	1
Lettuce	1
Tomato (1 medium)	1
Radish	1
Turnips	1

DAIRY & NUT MILKS

(1 cup)	PROTEIN IN GRAMS
Soy Milk	6 to 9
Almond Milk	1 to 2
Rice Milk	1
Eggs (1) (free-range)	6

FRUITS

(1 Serving or 1 cup)	PROTEIN IN GRAMS
Avocado (1 medium)	4
Banana (1)	1 to 2
Blackberries (1 cup)	2
Pomegranate (1)	1.5
Blueberries (1 cup)	1
Cantaloupe (1 cup)	1
Cherries (1 cup)	1
Grapes (1 cup)	1
Honeydew (1 cup)	1
Kiwi (1 large)	1
Lemon (1)	1
Mango (1)	1
Nectarine (1)	1
Orange (1)	1
Peach (1)	1
Pear (1)	1
Pineapple (1 cup)	1
Plum (1)	1
Raspberries (1 cup)	1
Strawberries (1 cup)	1
Watermelon (1 cup)	1

GRAINS & RICE

(1 cup cooked)	PROTEIN IN GRAMS
Triticale	25
Millet	8.4
Kamut	11
Amaranth	7
Oat Bran	7
Wild Rice	7
Couscous (whole wheat)	6
Bulgar Wheat	6
Buckwheat	6
Teff	6
Oat Groats	6
Barley	5
Quinoa	5
Brown Rice	5
Spelt	5

This chart displays the protein content of common vegetarian foods.
Note that in order to determine the amount of protein that is optimal for your body,
use the following formula that is based on a vegan diet: *the RDA recommends that
we take in 0.36 grams of protein per pound that we weigh* (100 lbs. x 0.36 = 36 grams).

Data from webs: *TheHolyKale.com • VegParadise.com • vrg.org (Vegetarian Resource Group).*

And what about that myth that you have to eat meat to get your protein? If that were true, where do you suppose farm animals, especially work horses and fast race horses get their protein? They are vegetarians! They get their protein from the grains and grasses that they eat. You are no different. You can get proteins you need from a large variety of organic whole grains, beans, raw nuts, seeds, fruits and vegetables that God put on this planet for your health and enjoyment!

We enjoy being vegetarians and not polluting our bodies with unhealthy meat, fowl and fish proteins. We feel it's safer and healthier getting proteins from organic vegetables, sprouts, beans, brown rice, legumes, nuts, seeds, etc. See Vegetable Protein % Chart, previous page.

Unhealthy Diet Depletes Minerals in Body

Unbalanced and unhealthy diets can deplete body of calcium, magnesium, potassium and other major elements (page 162). Diets high in proteins, meats, fish, and eggs may provide excess phosphorus which depletes calcium and magnesium from bones and tissues. This causes these minerals to be lost in the urine. High fat diets tend to increase uptake of phosphorus from intestines relative to calcium and other basic minerals. High phosphorus diet sodas can also produce losses of calcium, magnesium, etc.

Deficiencies of calcium and magnesium can produce many different health problems, from osteoporosis to muscular cramping, hyperactivity, muscular twitching (Restless Leg Syndrome effects millions), sleep disorders and frequency of urination. Deficiencies or imbalances of other minerals can produce many other health problems.

It is very important to clean and detoxify the body through fasting and by drinking 8 glasses pure distilled water and organically grown vegetable and fruit juices. In order to continually provide the body with new supplies of minerals, adults need a diet containing a variety of organic vegetables, also mineral rich kelp and other sea vegetables. Also infants need healthy mother's milk preferably to one year of age and longer when possible for solid foundation!

I live on legumes, vegetables & fruits. No dairy, no meat of any kind, no chicken, no turkey, & very little fish, once in a while. It changed my metabolism & I lost 24 pounds. I did research & found 82% of people who go on a plant-based diet begin to heal themselves, as I did. – U.S. President Bill Clinton, 1993-2001

Many adults and children in western civilizations are malnourished and have low levels of essential minerals in their bodies due to losses caused by consuming coffee, tea, cola and carbonated beverages and processed foods and modern diets containing refined flours, sugar and salt.

The body's organ systems can become so unbalanced by chronic stress; by toxins in our air, water and soil; by disease-produced injuries; and in babies, by prenatal nutritional deficiencies in the mother's diet and their unhealthy lifestyle habits! Thus, people in our fast-food society wisely need natural multi-vitamin and mineral food supplements to ensure they get their vital nutrients. We suggest everyone take them for extra protection.

Do Not Poison Your Body with Unhealthy, Toxic, Foodless Foods and Harmful Drinks!

In our industrialized, urbanized civilization, we pay a heavy price for the convenience of mass distribution of foodstuffs. Not only has our flour been bleached and robbed of its vital wheat germ, but the majority of commercial foods have been devitalized, demineralized – rendered foodless – in order to give them a longer shelf life! You are risking your own life when you eat these foodless foods that cannot nourish your body properly! Many contain preservatives and additives (such as nitrates and nitrites) whose cumulative effect has proven to be extremely harmful to the human body.

Even though the Federal Food & Drug Administration (FDA) requires label listing of ingredients on processed, packaged and canned foods, few people bother to read label fine print. If they do, they rarely understand it or take the trouble to find out what the various additives are and what effect they have on the human body! You don't have to be a chemist to find answers; just *Google* or look in modern dictionary.

Healthy Snack Munching: *Teenagers do a lot of their snacking and eating away from home, buying food from theaters, vending machines, fast-food outlets, shopping mall food courts, etc. But when armed with right health guidance from parents and healthy school food programs, they can wisely select and be satisfied with healthy choices: fruits & juice drinks, whole grain & honey bakery items rather than high-fat, sugared, white flour snacks that are mostly void of nutrition, and harmful to health, plus can cause weight gain, diabetes and obesity.*

Love, kindness and compassion are necessities, not luxuries . . . without them humanity cannot survive. – The Dalai Lama, Bragg Liquid Aminos Fan

Avoid All Dangerous Embalmers & Preservatives

For example, *Webster's Dictionary* defines **nitrate** as a *"salt or ester of nitric acid"* and defines **nitric acid** as a *"corrosive liquid inorganic acid HNO3"*. Ordinary common sense can figure out what a steady diet of toxic foods containing a concentrated form of a corrosive liquid inorganic acid will do to your body! **Nitrates and nitrites are deadly preservatives. Avoid them like the plague!**

Sulphur dioxide is another commercial preservative commonly used on dried fruits. It is defined by Webster as a *"heavy pungent gas, easily condensed to a colorless liquid and used especially in making sulfuric acid."* Do we have to remind you that sulfuric acid eats away flesh?

Many natural fats and oils are ruined by *hydrogenation.* This toxic hardening process keeps them from becoming rancid, but renders them absolutely indigestible and can cause terrible clogging of the cardiovascular system. Read all labels and understand them! Stop eating all commercially refined and processed foods made with refined white flour, refined white sugar, processed *lunch meats* and cheeses and foods with hydrogenated fats, harmful additives and many preservatives such as sodium nitrate, MSG (monosodium glutamate), sulfur dioxide, etc.

Although they are not labeled a *poison,* coffee, tea and alcohol should be banished from your diet! Why? Because their harmful ingredients accumulate poisons in your body. Also avoid soft drinks and cola drinks! They contain toxic fluoridated water, artificial flavors, colors, preservatives and sweeteners. They will slowly poison your bloodstream and body. The huge quantities of phosphorus in soda depletes calcium and magnesium from the body. Result: millions suffer with osteoporosis.

Just one caffeinated drink – a soft drink, caffeinated tea or coffee, will put your body on the caffeine roller-coaster. Caffeine doesn't provide energy to your system, it just burns up your reserves faster. You get a short-term boost at expense of long-term jitters and fatigue. When adrenal coffee high wears off, you feel drop in terms of fatigue, irritability, mood swings, depression, headache or confusion. – Stephen Cherniske, "Caffeine Blues"– Amazon.com

---

Caffeine depletes body of Vitamin B, which you need for proper brain and nervous system functioning and for converting food to energy. – Michael T. Murray, ND, Author "Getting Well Naturally – Chronic Fatigue Syndrome" – Amazon.com

Avoid These Processed, Refined, Harmful Foods

Once you realize the harm caused to your body by unhealthy, refined, chemicalized, deficient foods, you'll want to eliminate these "killer" foods! Also avoid microwaved foods! Follow The Bragg Healthy Lifestyle to provide the basic, healthy nourishment to maintain your health.

- Refined sugar, artificial sweeteners (toxic aspartame) in these products such as jams, jellies, preserves, marmalades, yogurts, ice cream, sherbets, Jello, cake, candy, cookies, all chewing gum, colas & diet drinks, pies, pastries, & all sugared fruit juices & fruits canned in sugar syrup. (**Health Stores have delicious healthy replacements for you, such as Stevia, raw honey, 100% maple syrup and agave nectar.**)

- White flour products such as white bread, wheat-white bread, enriched flours, rye bread that has white flour in it, dumplings, biscuits, buns, gravy, pasta, pancakes, waffles, soda crackers, pizza, ravioli, pies, pastries, cakes, cookies, prepared & commercial puddings & ready-mix bakery products. Most are made with dangerous (oxy-cholesterol) powdered milk & powdered eggs. (**Health Stores have huge variety of 100% whole grain organic products, delicious breads, crackers, pastas, desserts, etc.**)

- Salted foods, as salted potato chips, corn chips, pretzels, crackers & nuts.

- Refined white rice & pearl barley. • Fried fast foods. • Indian ghee.

- Refined, sugared (also aspartame) dry processed cereals – cornflakes, etc.

- Foods that contain Olestra, BakeLean, palm & cottonseed oil. These are not fit for human consumption & should be totally avoided.

- Peanuts & peanut butter that contain hydrogenated, hardened oils & any peanuts with mold. Molds can cause allergies & respiratory problems.

- Margarine – combines heart-deadly trans-fatty acids and saturated fats.

- Saturated fats & hydrogenated oils – enemies that clog the arteries.

- Coffee – even decaffeinated & caffeinated (in some green) teas & alcohol. Also all caffeinated and sugared water-juices, all cola and soft drinks.

- Fresh pork and products. • Fried, fatty, greasy meats. • Irradiated, GMO foods.

- Smoked meats, such as ham, bacon, sausage & smoked fish.

- Luncheon meats, hot dogs, salami, bologna, corned beef, pastrami & packaged meats containing dangerous sodium nitrate or nitrite.

- Dried fruits containing sulphur dioxide – a toxic preservative.

- Don't eat chickens or turkeys that have been injected with hormones or fed with commercial poultry feed containing any drugs or toxins.

- Canned soups – read labels for sugar, salt, starch, flour & preservatives.

- Foods containing benzoate of soda, salt, sugar, cream of tartar & any additives, drugs, preservatives; irradiated & genetically engineered foods.

- Day-old cooked vegetables, potatoes & pre-mixed, wilted lifeless salads.

- All commercial vinegars: pasteurized, filtered, distilled, white, malt & synthetic vinegars are dead vinegars! (*We use only Bragg Organic Raw, unfiltered Apple Cider Vinegar with the "Mother Enzyme" as used in olden times.*)

Modern GMO Wheat – No Longer Mother Nature's Wheat!!!

Modern GMO wheat isn't really the wheat that Mother Nature intended. About 700 million tons of wheat are grown worldwide making it second most-produced grain after corn. It's grown on more land area than any other commercial crop and considered a staple food for humans.

The Wheat We Eat Today Isn't the Wheat Our Grandmothers Ate!

The balance and ratio of nutrients that "Mother Nature" created for wheat has been modified! At some point in our history, this ancient grain was nutritious, however modern GMO wheat really isn't the same wheat at all. Once agribusiness took over to develop a higher-yielding crop, wheat became hybridized to the extent it has completely transformed from its prehistorical genetic configuration.

The majority of wheat is processed into 60% extraction or bleached white flour. The standard for most wheat products means that 40% of the original wheat grain is removed! So not only do we have an unhealthier, modified, and hybridized strain of wheat, we also remove and further degrade its nutritional value by processing it!

Unfortunately, the 40% that gets removed includes the bran and the germ of the wheat grain – its most nutrient-rich parts. In the process of making 60% extraction flour, most of the vitamin B1, B2, B3, E, folic acid, calcium, phosphorus, zinc, copper, iron, and fiber sadly are lost. **Any processed foods with GMO wheat are unhealthy since they cause more body health risks than benefits.**

Heavily marketed white carbs (white sugar, flour, pasta, etc.) that are packaged in boxes are designed to make you crave more. They're not good for your body, your mind or your soul! – BetterNutrition.com

Seek out, and choose healthy whole foods: organic fruits, vegetables, rice, beans, nuts, seeds, etc. rather than commercial, refined white flour and sugar products and highly processed canned goods in center aisles.

People who turn away from GMO wheat have dropped substantial weight. Even diabetics no longer become diabetic; people with arthritis have dramatic relief; and less acid reflux; leg swelling; and irritable bowel syndrome.

"The whiter the bread, the sooner you're dead!"
The body doesn't recognize processed GMO wheat as food. Nutrient absorption from processed wheat products is thus consequential with almost no nutritional value.

Even if you choose 100% whole wheat products they are based on modern GMO wheat strains created by irradiation of wheat seeds and embryos with chemicals, gamma rays, and high-dose X-rays to induce mutations. You're still consuming genetically modified grain.

To avoid all the toxic GMO wheat-oriented products, eat healthy foods – organic nuts, fruits and vegetables along with products made with non-GMO organic grains.

Health Problems Associated With GMO Wheat

Dr. Marcia Alvarez who specializes in nutritional programs for obese patients says, "**Modern GMO wheat grains could certainly be considered as the root of all evil in the world of nutrition** since they cause so many documented health problems across so many populations in the world." **See web:** *NonGMOproject.org*

Dr. Alvarez asserted that modern GMO wheat is now responsible for more intolerances than almost any other food in the world! "In my practice of over two decades, we have documented that for every ten people with digestive problems, obesity, irritable bowel syndrome, diabetes, arthritis and even heart disease, 8 out of 10 people have health problems with wheat! Once we remove modern GMO wheat from their diets, most of their symptoms disappear within 3 to 6 months," she added. Dr. Alvarez estimates that between coming influx of genetically modified (GMO) strains of wheat and current growing tendency of wheat elimination worldwide, that a trend is emerging in the next 20 years that will likely see 80% of people stop their consumption of GMO wheat in any form!

If you select 100% organic whole wheat products, the bran and germ of the wheat will remain in the product, and the health benefits will be impressive! Organic non-GMO whole wheat is a good dietary fiber source. – WHFoods.com

---

Food fiber is vital for good health, healthy elimination and adequate intake helps prevent colon cancer! Everyone should benefit from making sure they regularly include in their diet foods such as organic non-GMO whole grains, barley, oats, beans, fruits and vegetables that provide healthy food fibers.

Caution Using Salt – It's a Slow Killer!

We can't stress it enough: Avoid using salt!

The *salt of the earth* (inorganic sodium chloride) is poisonous to humans, plants and animals. What about *salt licks?* Don't even wild animals crave salt? My father investigated this thoroughly – and found that salt licks never contain sodium chloride. They are decomposed plant life made into organic minerals. Commercial salt licks used by cattle ranchers are to make cattle thirsty so they will drink volumes of water (like bars give free pretzels). Cattle weigh more (means more money) when ready to be sold. This is why meat *shrinks* excessively when cooked.

Salt was the first food preservative discovered by man. Remember, they had no refrigeration or means of storing food for long periods. Because their lifestyles were extremely active, their bodies could eliminate this indigestible salt, an inorganic mineral that plays havoc in the body. They stayed healthy until introduced to western diet poisons! Then their deterioration is rapid and tragic. My father and I have seen this especially in the South Sea islands, Hawaii, Samoa and Tahiti!

Most civilized people over 40, today are sedentary creatures. Most cannot eliminate or assimilate the excessive amount of salt they eat. Their bodies stash it away in crystals that harden in the artery lining and blood vessels and in joints, feet and hands, etc. causing arthritis and pain! Some salt is stored in a water solution that bloats the tissues. This can cause congestive heart failure and even death. Eliminate salt from your diet! *I occasionally use Himalyan Salt if needed. – PB.* If you think your food tastes *flat* without it, add Bragg Aminos, Bragg Kelp, or our delicious organic Bragg Sprinkle (24 herbs & spices) seasoning. Learn from famous French chefs, who use very little or no salt! They achieve marvelous flavors by skillful use of herbs, garlic, onions and mushrooms. Also Bragg Vinegar and lemon juice are good seasoners for salads, veggies, beans, rice, and legumes, etc.

Salt actually deadens your taste buds. Stay away from salt – we do! Your taste buds will awaken and soon start to enjoy the natural flavors of foods you eat. Even more importantly, you will become healthier and live longer when you give up salt and live a 100% healthy lifestyle!

Too much salt can cause high blood pressure, edema & kidney stones, etc.

8 Glasses Pure Water – Essential for Health!

Distilled water is the world's purest and best water! It's excellent for detoxification and fasting programs because it helps cleanse and flush toxins and harmful substances out of the body cells, organs and fluids of the body!

Most water from chemically-treated (toxic fluorides, chlorides, etc.) public water systems, and even some wells and springs, most likely contain harmful chemicals and toxic elements. Too often the water in our homes, offices, schools, hospitals, etc., are loaded with toxins; zinc, copper, cadmium or even lead from old soldered pipes.

The pure water from the fresh juices of vegetables, fruits and other foods, or the clean rain (distilled) water or steam (bottled) distilled water is essential for super health! Your body is constantly working for you. Your body is 70% water. The liquids you put in it will either nourish you or harm you, may even eventually kill you!

Your body constantly breaks down old bone and tissue cells and replaces them with new ones! As your body casts off old minerals and broken-down cells, it must obtain new supplies of essential elements in order to make healthy, new cells! (Important reason to eat healthy foods.)

Scientists discovered that many disorders, including dental problems, different types of arthritis, osteoporosis and some forms of hardening of the arteries are in part due to imbalances in the levels and ratios of minerals in the body. Every body requires a proper balance of all the nutritive elements in order to remain healthy. It's as bad for a person to have too much of one item as it is to have too little of another. In order for calcium to be able to create new cells of bone and teeth, you must have adequate levels of phosphorus and magnesium. Yet, if there is too much of these minerals or too little calcium, etc. in the diet, old bone will be taken away, but new bone will not be formed. Read more info page 162.

The power of pure distilled water is the vital chemistry of life!

Distilled Water is the #1 Health Drink

Not merely on fast days, but every day of your life, let the water you drink be pure distilled water. You'll be *drinking oxygen* with this pure H_2O! As well as fresh fruit and vegetable juices – which are naturally distilled – this is the only *safe* water to drink on our polluted planet.

Even rain water – which is naturally distilled water when it leaves the clouds – is contaminated if it passes through a heavily polluted atmosphere. (We love the smell of rain-washed air.) Mineral water and ground water (from springs, wells, streams, etc.) contain inorganic minerals which cannot be assimilated by the body and which can collect in the body and produce harmful deposits in the blood vessels, joints, kidneys and gallbladder. Water from reservoirs chemically treated to kill germs contains inorganic minerals and harsh chemicals (toxic chlorine, etc.) that are very harmful to the body! Don't drink water treated by water softeners! It contains suspended inorganic minerals that produce more *suds* ideal for washing clothes and dishes; but this chemically softened water is harmful to your body.

Use distilled water for drinking and cooking to ensure a longer life and health for you and your family! You will find complete, documented reports on the web on health hazards of chemicalized, fluoride waters and reasons for drinking only pure distilled water in our book, *Water – The Shocking Truth!* (See book list pages 237-239 of this book.)

Protest - Keep Toxic Fluoride Out of Your Water

Most of the water that Americans drink has fluoride in it, including tap, bottled and canned drinks! Now, the ADA (American Dental Association) is insisting the FDA mandates the addition of fluoride to all bottled waters! Defend your right to drink pure, non-fluorited tap and bottled water! Challenge and stop local and state water fluoridation policies! Please write, fax or e-mail your state officials, Congressional representatives and the President! (*firstgov.gov*)

CHECK FOLLOWING WEBSITES FOR FLUORIDE UPDATES:

- *www.fluoridealert.org* • *www.keepers-of-the-well.org* • *www.bruha.com/fluoride*
- *www.fluorideresearch.org* • *www.bragg.com* • *www.wholywater.com/fluoride.html*
- *www.fluoridation.com* • *www.dentalwellness4u.com/oralhealth/fluoride.html*

The 70% Watery Human

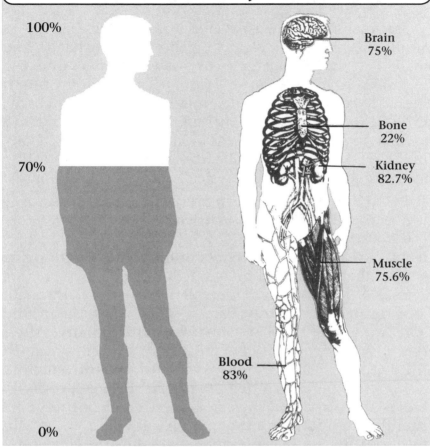

100%

70%

0%

Brain
75%

Bone
22%

Kidney
82.7%

Muscle
75.6%

Blood
83%

The amount of water in the human body, averaging 70%, varies considerably and even from one part of the body to another area as shown here. A lean man may hold 70% of his weight in body water, while a woman – because of her larger proportion of water-poor fatty tissues – may be only 52% water. The lowering of the water content in the blood is what triggers the hypothalamus, the brain's vital thirst center, to send out its familiar urgent demand for a drink of water! Please obey and drink ample amounts (8 glasses) of purified water daily. *By the time you feel thirsty, you're already dehydrated. – American Running & Fitness Association*

Water Percentage in Various Body Parts:

Teeth	10%	Spleen	75.5%
Bones	22%	Lungs	80%
Cartilage	55%	Blood	83%
Red blood corpuscles	68.7%	Bile	86%
Liver	71.5%	Plasma	90%
Brain	75%	Lymph	94%
Muscle tissue	75%	Saliva	95.5%

This chart shows why 8-10 glasses of pure water daily is so important.
Your body suffers when you're water dehydrated. The body's cells are like sponges. It takes time for cells to become hydrated. Daily drink 8 glasses of distilled water.

Juice Fast– Introduction to Water Fast

Fasting has been rediscovered, through juice fasting, as simple, easy means of cleansing and restoring health and vitality. To fast (*abstain from food, not water*) comes from Old English word *fasten* or *to hold firm*. It's a means to commit oneself to the task of finding inner strength through body, mind and soul cleansing. Throughout history the world's greatest philosophers and sages – including Socrates, Plato, Buddha, Gandhi and our Creator Jesus – practiced fasting and preached its great physical and spiritual benefits!

Juice bars are springing up everywhere and juice fasting has become *in* with the theatrical crowd in Hollywood, New York and London. The number of Stars who believe in the power and effectiveness of juice and water fasting is growing. A partial list includes: Steven Spielberg, Barbra Streisand, Kim Basinger, Alec Baldwin, Daryl Hannah, Christie Brinkley, Dolly Parton, Cloris Leachman and Donna Karan. They say fasting helps balance their lives physically, mentally, spiritually and emotionally. Although we feel a water fast is best, an introductory liquid juice fast can offer people an ideal opportunity to give their intestinal systems a restful, cleansing relief from the high fat, high sugar, high salt and high protein fast foods that so many Americans unhealthily exist on!

Organic, raw, live fruit and vegetable juices can be purchased fresh from Health Stores, farmer's markets and some super markets. You can also prepare healthy juices yourself using a home juicer. When juice fasting, it's best to dilute juice with 1/3 distilled water. The list on next page gives you many delicious combination ideas. With any vegetable and tomato combinations try adding a dash of Bragg Liquid Aminos, herbs or, on non-fast days, even some green powder (barley, chlorella, spirulina, etc.) to create a delicious, nutritious, powerful health drink! When using herbs in these drinks, use 1 to 2 fresh leaves or pinch of Bragg Sprinkle (24 herbs & spices) or Bragg Kelp (seaweed), rich in protein, iodine and iron is delicious with vegetable juices.

Fasting is an effective and safe method of detoxifying the body – a healing technique used for centuries. Fasting regularly one day a week can help the body cleanse and heal itself. Bragg Books were my conversion to the healthy way.
– James Balch, M.D. Co-Author of "Prescription for Nutritional Healing" – Amazon.com

Here's Some Powerful Juice Combinations:

1. Beet, celery, kale and carrots
2. Cabbage, celery and apple
3. Cabbage, cucumber, celery, tomato, kale, spinach and basil
4. Tomato, carrot and celery
5. Carrot, celery, kale garlic, watercress, blue or goji berries and wheatgrass
6. Grapefruit, orange and lemon
7. Beet, parsley, celery, carrot, mustard greens, cabbage, garlic
8. Beet, celery, kale and carrot
9. Cucumber, carrot and parsley
10. Watercress, apple, cucumber, garlic
11. Asparagus, carrot and apple
12. Carrot, celery, kale, parsley and cabbage, onion, sweet basil
13. Carrot, coconut milk and ginger
14. Carrot, broccoli, lemon, cayenne
15. Carrot, sprouts, kelp, rosemary
16. Apple, carrot, radish, ginger
17. Apple, pineapple and seaweed
18. Apple, papaya and grapes
19. Papaya, blueberries and apple
20. Leafy greens, broccoli, apple
21. Grape, apple and blueberries
22. Watermelon (best alone)

Paul C. Bragg Introduced Juicing to America

Juicing has come a long way since my father imported the first hand operated vegetable-fruit juicer from Germany. Before, this juice was pressed by hand using cheesecloth. He introduced his new juice therapy idea, then pineapple juice, then later tomato juice, to the American public. These two juices were erroneously thought to be too acid! Now, these health beverages have become the favorites of millions. TV's famous Juicemen Jack LaLanne and Jay Kordich say Bragg was their early inspiration and mentor! They both loved living The Bragg Healthy Lifestyle and inspiring millions to health.

LIQUEFY OR JUICE FRESH ORGANIC FRUITS & VEGETABLES

The juicer, food processor and blender are great for preparing foods, drinks, gentle (bland) diets and baby foods, etc. Fibers of juiced fresh fruits and vegetables can be tolerated on most gentle diets. Any raw or cooked fruit or vegetable can be liquefied and added to broth, soups and non-dairy (soy, rice or coconut) milks. Fresh juices supercharge your energy level and boost your immune system to maximize body's health power. You may fortify liquid meals or Bragg Smoothies with green vegetable powders, alfalfa, barley green, chlorella, spirulina and wheat grass for extra nutrition.

Fruit bears the closest relation to light. The sun pours a continuous flood of light into the fruits, and they furnish the best potion of food a human being requires for the sustenance of mind, body and life. – Louisa May Alcott, 1868

Increasing intake of fruits and vegetables can help you prevent heart disease, cancer and other chronic diseases. Surveys show those who increased their daily fruit and vegetable intake improved their health, vitality and well-being.
– UC Berkeley Wellness Letter • www.BerkeleyWellness.com

Organic whole grains, vegetables, fruits, raw nuts and seeds give needed vitamins and minerals to the body. – Patricia Bragg, ND, PhD., Health Crusader

Fast One Day Each Week for Inner Cleansing

Fasting is the greatest cleanser and body purifier. Give it a chance to do thorough house cleansing: help your body rid itself of accumulated toxic poisons by going on a 24 to 36 hour fast every week. Monday is our favorite fast day.

During this fast, drink 8-10 glasses of distilled water daily. Flavor with fresh lemon juice or 1-2 tsps Bragg Organic Raw Apple Cider Vinegar (ACV) with 1-2 tsps. (optional) honey, maple syrup to taste or diabetics can use drop or pinch of Stevia Herb. Some add pinch of cayenne. No food, juices or supplements are necessary. Some start with juice fasts pages 144-145. If you want warm drink, have herbal tea or delicious hot Bragg Liquid Aminos Broth (1 tsp in cup hot water) or Bragg Vinegar Drinks (for pic, etc. page 244 or recipe page 149).

When freed from daily chores of digesting and assimilating food, your body will use its oxygen-sparked energy to do a more thorough internal cleansing! After your first fast you will feel a renewed vitality. Make this a weekly habit and, as time goes on, you will feel even more invigorated and rejuvenated. Life is precious – Monday is our regular weekly fast day. After evening meal on Sunday, we take nothing but 8-10 glasses of distilled water (to 3 add 2 tsps. ACV) until Tuesday morning. The Bragg Family has been doing this fast for 90 years and are all living healthy, long lives. We also fast the first 3 days of each month. Several times each year we do longer fasts of 7-10 days. Our favorite fast is distilled water for a week. It works wonders in keeping us fit and trim. For more info about methods and benefits of fasting, consult our book, *The Miracle of Fasting*. Read page 147. (This book has changed the lives of millions worldwide. It's been #1 in Russia and the Ukraine for over 50 years.)

Oil Pulling May Transform Your Health

The ancient Ayurvedic remedy for oral health and detoxification is in oil pulling! It involves the use of pure oil – as organic olive oil, for pulling harmful bacteria, fungus and other organisms out of the mouth, teeth, gums and even throat. All you need to do is place about a tablespoon of oil into your mouth and swish it around for about 10-15 minutes, then please spit it out! Lipids in the oil pulls out toxins and the oil absorbs toxins and bacteria. The oil helps in cellular restructuring, proper functioning of lymph nodes and other internal organs. People write us of their great results using Bragg Organic Olive Oil. – OilPulling.com

146

⟨ BENEFITS FROM THE JOYS OF FASTING ⟩

Fasting renews your faith in yourself, your strength and God's strength.
Fasting is easier than any diet. • Fasting is the quickest way to lose weight.
Fasting is adaptable to a busy life. • Fasting gives the body a physiological rest.
Fasting is used successfully in the treatment of many physical illnesses.
Fasting can yield weight losses of up to 10 pounds or more in the first week.
Fasting lowers & normalizes cholesterol, homocysteine & blood pressure levels.
Fasting improves dietary habits. • Fasting increases pleasure eating healthy foods.
Fasting is a calming experience, often relieving tension and insomnia.
Fasting frequently induces feelings of happy euphoria, a natural high.
Fasting is a miracle rejuvenator, helps in slowing the ageing process.
Fasting is a natural stimulant to rejuvenate the growth hormone levels.
Fasting is an energizer, not a debilitator. • Fasting aids the elimination process.
Fasting often results in a more vigorous happy marital relationship.
Fasting can eliminate smoking, drug and drinking addictions.
Fasting is a regulator, educating the body to consume food only as needed.
Fasting saves precious time spent on marketing, preparing and eating.
Fasting rids the body of toxins, giving it an internal shower & cleansing.
Fasting does not deprive the body of essential nutrients.
Fasting can be used to uncover the sources of food allergies.
Fasting is used effectively in schizophrenia treatment & other mental illnesses.
Fasting under proper supervision can be tolerated easily up to four weeks.
Fasting does not accumulate appetite; hunger pangs disappear in 1-2 days.
Fasting is routine for most of the animal kingdom.
Fasting has been a common practice since the beginning of man's existence.
Fasting is practiced in all religions; the Bible alone has 74 references to fasting.
Fasting under proper conditions is absolutely safe. • Fasting is a blessing.

"Fasting As A Way Of Life" – Allan Cott, M.D.
Fasting is not starving, it's nature's cure that God has given us. – Patricia Bragg

Spiritual Bible Reasons Why We Should Fast

Acts 13:2-3	Neh. 1:4	Luke 4:2-5, 14	Deut. 8:3-8	Matthew 9:9-15
Acts 14:23-25	Ezra 8:21	Luke 9:1-6, 11	Joel 2:12	Matthew 17:18-21
3 John 2	Gal. 5:16-26	Mark 2:16-20	Matthew 7:7-8	Deut. 11:7-14, 21
1 Cor. 10:31	Gen. 6:3	Matthew 4:1-4	Psalms 119:18	Neh. 9:1, 20-21
1 Cor. 13:4-7	Isaiah 58:6,8	Psalms 69:11	Psalms 35:13	Matthew 6:16-18

Dear Health Friend,

This gentle reminder explains the great benefits from *The Miracle of Fasting* that you will enjoy when starting on your weekly 24 hour Bragg Fasting Program for Super Health! It's a precious time of body-mind-soul cleansing and renewal.

On fast days I drink 8-10 glasses of distilled (our favorite) or purified water, (I add 1-2 tsps Bragg Organic Vinegar to 3 of them). If just starting, you may also try herbal teas or try diluted fresh juices with 1/3 distilled water. Every day, even some fast days, add 1 Tbsp of psyllium husk powder to liquids once daily. It's an extra cleanser and helps normalize weight, cholesterol and blood pressure and helps promote healthy elimination. Fasting is the oldest, most effective healing method known to man. Fasting offers great miraculous blessings from Mother Nature and our Creator. It begins the self-cleansing of the inner-body workings so we can promote our own self-healing.

My father and I wrote the book *The Miracle of Fasting* to share with you the health miracles it can perform in your life. It's all so worthwhile to do and it's an important part of The Bragg Healthy Lifestyle.

With Love, *Patricia*

Paul Bragg's work on fasting and water is one of the great contributions to The Healing Wisdom and The Natural Health Movement in the world today.
– Gabriel Cousens, M.D., Author of "Conscious Eating" and "Spiritual Nutrition"

Food and Product Summary

Today, sadly many foods are highly processed or refined, robbing them of essential nutrients, vitamins, minerals and enzymes. Many also contain harmful, toxic and dangerous chemicals. The Research findings and experience of top Nutritionists, Physicians and Dentists have led to the discovery that devitalized foods are a major cause of poor health, illness, cancer and premature death! The enormous increase in the last 70 years of degenerative diseases such as heart disease, arthritis, diabetes and dental decay, etc. backs this belief. Scientific Research has shown most of these afflictions can be prevented and others, once established, can be arrested or even reversed through nutritional methods – page 131.

Enjoy Super Health with Natural Foods

1. **RAW FOODS:** Fresh fruits and raw vegetables organically grown are always best! Enjoy nutritious variety garden salads with raw vegetables, sprouts, raw nuts and seeds.

2. **VEGETABLES and PROTEINS:**
   a. Legumes, lentils, brown rice, soy beans, and all beans.
   b. Nuts and seeds, raw and unsalted.
   c. We prefer healthier vegetarian proteins. If you must have animal protein, then be sure it's hormone–free, and organically fed and no more than 1 or 2 times a week.
   d. Dairy products – fertile range-free eggs (*not over 4 weekly*), unprocessed hard cheese and feta goat's cheese. We choose not to use dairy products. Try the healthier non-dairy soy, rice, coconut, and almond milks and soy cheeses, delicious soy yogurt and soy and rice ice cream.

3. **FRUITS and VEGETABLES:** Organically grown is always best – grown without the use of poisonous sprays and toxic chemical fertilizers whenever possible; do urge your markets to stock healthier organic produce! Steam, bake, sauté and wok vegetables as short a time as possible to retain the best nutritional content and flavor. Also enjoy fresh juices.

4. **100% WHOLE GRAIN CEREALS, BREADS and FLOURS:** They contain important B-complex vitamins, vitamin E, minerals, fiber and the important unsaturated fatty acids.

5. **COLD or EXPELLER-PRESSED VEGETABLE OILS:** Bragg Organic First Press, Extra Virgin Olive Oil (is best), soy, flax, sunflower, and sesame oils are good sources of healthy, essential, unsaturated fatty acids. We still use oils sparingly.

HEALTHY BEVERAGES
Fresh Juices, Herb Teas & Energy Drinks

These freshly squeezed organic vegetable and fruit juices are important to The Bragg Healthy Lifestyle. It's not wise to drink beverages with your main meals, as it dilutes the digestive juices. But it's great during the day to have a glass of freshly squeezed orange, grapefruit, vegetable juice, Bragg Vinegar ACV Drink, herb tea or try hot cup Bragg Liquid Aminos Broth ($^1/_2$ to 1 tsp. Bragg Liquid Aminos in cup of hot distilled water) – these are all ideal pick-me-up beverages.

Bragg Apple Cider Vinegar Cocktail – Mix 1 to 2 tsps. Bragg Organic ACV and (*optional*) to taste raw honey, agave nectar or pure maple syrup (*if diabetic, to sweeten use 2 stevia drops*) in 8 oz. of distilled or purified water. Take glass upon arising, hour before lunch and dinner. Bragg Organic ACV drinks now available in 6 fruit flavors, see page 244.

Delicious Hot or Cold Cider Drink – Add 2 to 3 cinnamon sticks and 4 cloves to water and boil. Steep 20 minutes or more. Before serving add Bragg Vinegar and sweetener to taste (*Re-use cinnamon sticks & cloves*).

Bragg Favorite Juice Cocktail – This drink consists of all raw vegetables (remember organic is best) which we prepare in our juicer or blender: carrots, celery, beets, cabbage, tomatoes, watercress, kale, and parsley, etc. The great purifier, garlic we enjoy, but it's optional.

Bragg Favorite Healthy Energy Smoothie – After morning stretch and exercises we often enjoy this drink below instead of fruit. It's delicious and powerfully nutritious as a meal anytime: lunch, dinner or take in thermos to work, school, sports, gym, hiking, and to park or freeze for popsicles.

Bragg Healthy Energy Smoothie

Prepare following in blender, add frozen juice cubes if desired colder; Choice of: freshly squeezed orange or grapefruit juice; carrot and greens juice; unsweetened pineapple juice; or $1^1/_2$ - 2 cups purified or distilled water with:

2 tsps spirulina or green powder　　　*1 to 2 bananas, ripe*
$^1/_3$ tsp Bragg Nutritional Yeast　　　　*or fresh fruit in season*
2 dates or prunes-pitted　　　　　*1-2 tsps almond or nut butter*
1 "Emergen-C" Vitamin C packet　　*$^1/_2$ tsp lecithin granules*
1 tsp protein powder　　　　　　*1 tsp raw honey (optional)*
1 tsp flaxseed oil or grind seeds　　*$^1/_2$ tsp rice or oat bran*

Optional: 4-6 apricots (sun-dried,) soak in jar overnight in purified distilled water or unsweetened pineapple juice. We soak enough to last for several days. Keep refrigerated. In summer you can add organic fresh fruit: peaches, papaya, blueberries, strawberries, all berries, apricots, etc. instead of banana. In winter, add apples, kiwi, oranges, tangelos, persimmons or pears, and if the fresh is unavailable, try sugar-free, frozen organic fruits. Serves 1 to 2.

Patricia's Delicious Health Popcorn

Use freshly popped organic popcorn (use air popper). Try Bragg Organic Olive Oil or flaxseed oil or melted salt-free butter over popcorn and add several sprays of Bragg Liquid Aminos and Bragg Apple Cider Vinegar – Yes, it's delicious! Now sprinkle with Bragg Nutritional Yeast Seasoning and Bragg Sprinkle (24 herbs & spices). For a variety try a pinch of cayenne pepper, mustard powder or fresh crushed garlic to oil mixture. Serve instead of breads!

Bragg Lentil & Brown Rice Casserole, Burgers or Soup
Jack LaLanne's Favorite Recipe

16 oz pkg organic lentils, uncooked   4 garlic cloves, chop
1 cup brown organic rice, uncooked   2 onions, chop
5 cups, distilled / purified water   2 tsps Bragg Liquid Aminos
4 - 6 carrots, chop $^1/_2$" rounds   1 tsp Bragg Sprinkle (24 Herbs & Spices)
3 celery stalks, chop   2 tsps Bragg Organic Virgin Olive Oil
1 cup diced fresh or canned tomatoes (salt-free)

Wash & drain lentils & rice. Place grains in large stainless steel pot. Add water, bring to boil, reduce heat & simmer 30 minutes. Now add vegetables & Bragg Seasonings & cook on low heat until tender. Last 5 minutes add fresh or canned (salt-free) tomatoes. For delicious garnish, add minced parsley & Bragg Nutritional Yeast Seasoning. **For Burgers mash. For Soup, add more water in cooking grains.** Serves 4 to 6.

Bragg Raw Organic Vegetable Health Salad

2 stalks celery, chop $^1/_2$ cup red cabbage, chop
1 bell pepper & seeds, dice $^1/_2$ cup alfalfa or sunflower sprouts
$^1/_2$ cucumber, slice   2 spring onions & green tops, chop
2 carrots, grate   1 turnip, grate
1 raw beet, grate   1 avocado (ripe)
1 cup green cabbage, chop   3 tomatoes, medium size

For variety add organic raw zucchini, sugar peas, mushrooms, broccoli, cauliflower, (try black olives & pasta). Chop, slice or grate vegetables fine to medium for variety in size. Mix vegetables & serve on bed of lettuce, spinach, watercress or chopped cabbage. Dice avocado and tomato, serve in bowl as a dressing. Serve choice of fresh squeezed lemon, orange or dressing separately. Chill salad plates before serving. **It's best to always eat salad first before hot dishes.** Serves 3 to 5.

Bragg Health Salad Dressing

$^1/_2$ cup Bragg Organic Apple Cider Vinegar $^1/_2$ tsp Bragg Liquid Aminos
1-2 tsps organic raw honey   1-2 cloves garlic, minced
$^1/_3$ cup Bragg Organic Olive Oil, or blend with safflower, soy, sesame or flax oil
1 Tbsp fresh herbs, minced or pinch of Bragg Sprinkle (24 herbs & spices)

Blend ingredients in blender or jar. Refrigerate in covered jar.

FOR DELICIOUS HERBAL VINEGAR: In quart jar add $^1/_3$ cup tightly packed, crushed fresh sweet basil, tarragon, dill, oregano, or any fresh herbs desired, combined or singly (If *dried* herbs, use 1-2 tsps herbs). Now cover to top with Bragg Organic Apple Cider Vinegar and store two weeks in warm place, and then strain and refrigerate.

MY DAILY HEALTH JOURNAL

Today is:____/____/____

> *I have said my morning resolve and am ready to practice*
> *The Bragg Healthy Lifestyle today and every day.*

Yesterday I went to bed at: Today I arose at: Weight:

Today I practiced the No-Heavy Breakfast or No-Breakfast Plan: ☐ yes ☐ no

• For Breakfast I drank: Time:

   For Breakfast I ate:

      Time:

Supplements:

• For Lunch I ate: Time:

Supplements:

• For Dinner I ate: Time:

Supplements:

• ____ Glasses of Water I Drank during the Day, including ACV Drinks

   List Snacks – Kind and When:

• **I took part in these physical (walking, gym, etc.) activities today:**

Grade each on scale of 1 to 10 (desired optimum health is 10).

• **I rate my day for the following categories:**

Previous Night's Sleep:	Stress/Anxiety:
Energy Level:	Elimination:
Physical Activity, Exercise:	Health:
Peacefulness:	Accomplishments:
Happiness:	Self-Esteem:

• **General Comments, Reactions and To Do List:**

BRAGGZYME ®

SUPERIOR SYSTEMIC ENZYMES
Support for joints, muscles and immune system
FOR HEALTHY ACTIVE LIFESTYLE AND HEART SUPPORT

Dr. Paul C. Bragg, Health Pioneer, was the first to introduce enzyme supplements in Health Stores in 1931. Now Bragg Health Science Formulas are proud to introduce most advanced Systemic Enzyme Supplement available today. BRAGGZYME – Superior Systemic Enzyme, an all natural superior Systemic Fibrinolytic Enzyme that contains powerful 500mg Complex – Nattokinase, Serrapeptase, Bromelain, Papain, Protease, Lipase & CoQ10, with 4,500 Fibrinolytic Units (FU) per vegetable capsule.

"Good Circulation is Key to A Healthy Body!" – Paul C. Bragg, ND, PhD.

This exclusive systemic enzyme blend provides nutritional and cardiovascular support you need to help maintain a normal inflammatory response and maintain safe normal fibrin levels for a healthy cardiovascular system.* Braggzyme contains no animal derivatives, no artificial flavors, no artificial coloring, no yeast and no wheat.

- Enzyme support for back, joint, muscle, tendon and immune health system.*
- Boost energy levels – infuses life-giving oxygen to every cell in your body.*
- Nutritional support to help maintain a normal inflammatory response.*
- Helps eliminate dangerous fibrin levels for a healthier blood flow.*
- Helps keep your hands, feet and the entire body warm.*
- Helps improve and keep memory and brain sharp.*
- Contains no animal derivatives, no yeast, no wheat, no artificial flavors and no artificial colors.
- Kosher Certified.
- 100% Safe, All Natural Veg. Formula in Veg. Cap.

120 Veg Caps

* These statements have not been evaluated by the Food and Drug Administration. This product is not intended to diagnose, treat, cure, or prevent any disease.

"I have been taking Braggzyme for the last several months, and have felt a major improvement in my knee pain caused by sports, snowboarding, etc. Thanks, Braggzyme!"
– Brian Evans, Manager, Lassens Natural Foods, California

My doctor said that elevated fibrinogen levels are associated with an increased risk of heart attack and strokes because it can promote formation of dangerous blood clots. Good news! Since taking Braggzyme my fibrinogen level was 329 and now it's a safe 279. – Kathy Duerr, Oregon

Since on Braggzyme, I have great energy and no more body aches, pains and my memory is sharper. Thanks to Braggzyme. – R.J. DeCastro, California

Daily, upon awakening, I take 3 Braggzyme. – Patricia Bragg, ND, PhD.

Chapter 18

The Power of Vitamins

Eating Healthy Organic Foods Gives You More Nutrients, Super Oxygen, Energy and Health

Organic vegetables, fruits and grains are rich in nutrients and vitamins and contain large amounts of life-giving oxygen! Their juices are very rich in oxygen and distilled water which is Mother Nature's purest liquid!

Organic green leafy vegetables also supply organic iron, copper and other important vital minerals that are needed to manufacture hemoglobin in red blood cells. These enable the blood to absorb oxygen from the lungs and transport it to every part of your entire body.

Some cooked foods (grains, legumes, potatoes, vegetables, etc.) enhance a well-balanced healthy diet. Cooking can reduce, and in some cases, even eliminate the vitamin content. Don't overcook! We suggest you lightly steam, bake, broil, stir-fry or wok foods that need some cooking.

Vitamins That Help the Respiratory System

Vitamins play a vital role in keeping our respiratory system healthy and helps in reducing risk of diseases, such as **chronic obstructive pulmonary disease (COPD), emphysema, bronchitis, pneumonia and asthma.** Chronic lower respiratory diseases are the fourth leading cause of death in the U.S. If you are considering taking vitamins that can help with respiratory problems, talk with your health doctor first to determine best course of action.

Organic, non-GMO whole grain products are excellent sources of natural vitamin E, magnesium, selenium and vital nutrients important for maintaining a healthy heart and strong bones. Shocking studies found over 80% of nutrients are lost in refining grains into white flour!

Taking natural vitamins, minerals, trace minerals and herbs are healthy added insurance to help meet the bodies daily supplemental needs.

Studies show Vitamin C and E help alleviate severity of asthma symptoms.
– Life Extension Magazine (www.lef.org)

Vitamin A – for Healthy Respiratory System

Vitamin A is a fat soluble vitamin. It has an essential role in stimulating your immune system and fighting infections. Vitamin A also assists in maintaining normal vital lung function. It repairs and strengthens mucous membranes lining the lungs. Vitamin A maintains normal functioning of mucous membrane cells that protect the lungs from harmful airborne pathogens. Individuals with lung issues that hamper breathing can benefit by increasing vitamin A intake. (See web: *LiveStrong.com*)

Vitamin A deficiency can be damaging to the lungs, as revealed through animal testing and studies. Vitamin A deficiency can also increase your risk of respiratory infections. Research has revealed that the lower the Vitamin A in umbilical cord blood at the time of birth, the higher the risk of lower respiratory tract infections in preschool children between under 1 month to 5 years of age.

Folate and B Vitamins Boosts Immune System

Folate is a water soluble B vitamin that stimulates DNA production and cell reproduction. A folate deficiency can lead to an increase in risk of respiratory diseases and infections. Researchers found that folate deficiency in young children is an independent risk factor for lower respiratory tract infections. These Scientists also discovered that children who are breastfed have a lower risk of folate deficiency and respiratory tract infections.

Our body depends on vitamin B12 to produce healthy red blood cells (RBCs). Inadequate vitamin B12 lowers RBC count, a condition called anemia, that often leads to fatigue and breathing problems, which aggravates while exercising. RBCs perform the important job of delivering oxygen to each and every cell in the body. No wonder, vitamin B12 deficiency reduces oxygen flow to the body, resulting in shortness of breath. So, its intake may help to overcome breathing problems. Other Studies have shown that adequate levels of vitamin B6 in the blood can improve breathing, as well as significantly reduce the risk of lung cancer (*www.health.harvard.edu*).

Vitamin C Reduces Inflammation

Vitamin C – water soluble vitamin that stimulates immune system and protects cells from harmful substances. Increasing dietary intake of vitamin C helps reduce risk of respiratory infections. Studies report vitamin C supplementation can reduce common cold by 45-91%, and helps lower incidence of pneumonia by 80-100%.

Vitamin C can help reduce tightening of air passages, that usually happens during or shortly after exercising. This condition referred to as exercise-induced bronchoconstriction (EIB) causes airways to become inflamed, thereby restricting free air flow into the lungs. EIB is typically marked by coughing, wheezing, and breathing trouble! Study suggests vitamin C reduces inflammatory response, that contributes alleviating EIB.

Vitamin D – Improves Exercising Performance

Supplemental dosage of vitamin D plays a crucial role in enhancing respiratory muscle function and exercise performance in COPD patients! These patients were able to exercise with more vigor and intensity due to vitamin D. Even exercising for a short duration makes these patients gasp for breath. However, increasing the vitamin D intake helps COPD patients improve their breathing and exercise performance (pages 155-157, 182).

Sunshine Vitamin D3 – Essential for Health

Vital vitamin D3 is a natural hormone and like other hormones it's manufactured in the body. It helps body utilize calcium and phosphorus to build bones and teeth. Vitamin D3 also helps skin heal and boosts immune system. Statistics from a California survey of American women found women with higher sun exposure and those with a high dietary intake of vitamin D3, had a lower risk of breast cancer. Evidence also points to a link between vitamin D3 and reduced risk of colon cancer and bone fractures.

Skin produces approx 10,000 IUs of Vitamin D3 in response to 20-30 minutes in gentle sun exposure without using sunblock lotions.

There is evidence supporting the near-miraculous healing power of Vitamin D3, a nutrient that is available free just by enjoying gentle sunlight on your skin. Small amounts of gentle sunlight on your skin cells causes them to manufacture vitamin D3. Even as little as 10 to 20 minutes, 2 to 3 times a week should be sufficient to meet your needs. Sunscreen can reduce or even shut down the synthesis of vitamin D3, so we recommend exposure to gentle early morning or late afternoon rays without use of sunscreen! People under 50 years need 1,000 IUs, 50-70 years need 2,000 IUs and those over 70 need 2,000-5,000 IUs of vitamin D3 daily, more in special cases. Older people's ability to produce vitamin D3 from sunlight declines. That's why it's important for those over 70 to get vitamin D3 from supplements and foods: wheat germ, raw sunflower seeds, cod liver oil, sweet potatoes, corn bread, eggs, alfalfa, saltwater fish, sardines, salmon, tuna, liver and natural vegetable oils are good sources of vitamin D3.

An analysis of more that 15,000 Americans, those with low blood levels of Vitamin D3, were 30% more likely to have high blood pressure, 40% more apt too have high triglycerides, 98% more likely to be diabetic and 129% more apt to be obese! Researchers noted that low Vitamin D3 may also be a culprit for Fibromyalgia, Multiple Sclerosis, Rheumatoid Arthritis and other joint diseases.

Vitamin D3 is major protective factor guarding against chemical sensitivities and infections. Cod liver oil which parents once gave automatically to children is an excellent preventive medicine, with high concentrations of vitamins A & D3.
– Dr. Michael Schachter, Columbia University • www.mbschachter.com

---

Vitamin D3 is made when UVB light from the sun is absorbed by the skin. This is the most natural form. Most supplements sold today are Vitamin D3 (animal source – lanolin) or Vitamin D2 (fungus/yeast derived) ideal for vegetarians/vegans. Vitamin D3 is the more potent form of Vitamin D and has a better stable shelf-life. Learn more by reading "Vitamin D Solution" by Michael F. Holick, PhD, MD. Professor Boston University and recipient of prestigious "Linus Pauling Prize" for his extensive research on Vitamin D.

Magnesium may help vitamin D by activating vitamin D into a form your body can use. Magnesium is also important in helping vitamin D to maintain calcium in the body and is essential for bone health. Zinc also helps vitamin D to work inside the cells of your body. Vitamin D and zinc work together to strengthen your bones and to help them develop properly. – VitaminDcouncil.org

Five Ways Vitamin D3 Can Save Your Life

1. **Promotes Weight Loss:** You need Vitamin D3 to effectively help you lose weight. Your insulin works better and Vitamin D3 helps you lose belly fat. Diabetes is also related to low Vitamin D3 levels.
2. **Reduces Risk of Early, Pre-mature Death.**
3. **Fewer Bone Fractures**: Without Vitamin D3, calcium can't be absorbed. But if you get enough vitamin D3, it can help you avoid osteoporosis, bone fractures and falling, which is a cause of death among the elderly.
4. **Reduces Risk of Heart Disease:** Vitamin D3 improves blood flow by relaxing blood vessels and lowering blood pressure. (*We enjoy sunshine Vitamin D3! – PB.*)
5. **Helps Fight Cancer:** D3 improves the functioning of your immune system and that helps fight cancer!

Five Ways To Get Vitamin D3

1. **15 minutes of high-noon sun exposure** in warmer climates few times a week. (*We prefer early or late sun.*)
2. **Fatty Fish and Cod Liver Oil:** If you have been warned to stay out of the sun, another good source Vitamin D3 is oily fish, such as salmon, tuna, mackerel and trout.
3. **Fortified Dairy Products** (*We prefer soy non-dairy. – PB.*)
4. **Multi-Vitamin Supplements**: Most all multi-vitamins have a substantial amount of vitamin D3.
5. **Vitamin D Supplements:** 1000 to 2000 IUs Vitamin D3 recommended daily (*seniors 2000 - 3000 IUs, page 156*).

Taken from: "Good Morning America" – abcnews.go.com/GMA

Vitamin E – A Powerful Antioxidant

Vitamin E provides significant protective effects against wide range of respiratory disorders, including COPD. Taking vitamin E can help repair lung tissue and even rebuild lung capacity, in turn contributing to ease any breathing problems. Vitamin E also protects the lungs by nullifying the impact of inhaled pollutants. The possibility of using vitamin E as an *antidote to smog* has been well researched –

Good news about organic fruits & vegetables just won't stop! New study states high consumption of antioxidants – vitamin C, E, selenium and beta carotene improves lung function. These antioxidants also help improve lung function and protect against Chronic Obstructive Pulmonary Disease (COPD). – DrMercola.com

Dr. Al L. Tappel, Biochemistry Professor, University of California, Davis, states that the natural antioxidation property of vitamin E helps reverse the ageing process. He recommends vitamin E supplements for everyone to help promote a healthier, longer life. *For more suggestions on natural supplements and herbs read pages 33, 38, 162 and 182.*

Add Wonder-Working Vitamin E Tocotrienols

E Tocotrienols provide greater antioxidant protection against lipid peroxidation than standard vitamin E. This oxygen conserving ability of vitamin E Tocotrienols may be effective in relief of emphysema, the deadly disease of lung deterioration which has increased as our air has become more contaminated. Another vitamin E healing gift is its oil as an amazingly effective skin treatment for home application to minor burns, sunburn, skin rashes, scars, and even stretch marks (from pregnancy).

Miracle natural vitamin E Tocotrienols supplements are available at health stores. If just starting vitamin E, doctors recommend you begin with 100 IUs daily. Gradually increase to 800 IUs for women and 1200 IUs for men. Raw wheat germ flakes (vacuum packed) and its oil are good sources (page 160). Refrigerate both after opening!

Raw wheat germ (high in vitamin E) perishes easily. That is why it is refined out of white flour. Apparently the commercial millers are more interested in the shelf life of their product, than in the length of your life.

In Bragg household, we often sprinkle raw wheat germ flakes over raw garden salads, potatoes, vegetables, soups, etc. It has a pleasant, nutty taste. If you like the taste of wheat germ oil (some do, some don't), you can add some to salad dressings. Parents can even add wheat germ oil to baby's soy, nut or Rice Dream milk. Hollywood Clint Eastwood's children thrived on wheat germ oil added to goat's milk ($^1/_4$ tsp. per cup) after being weaned at one year.

Vitamin E protects cells from damaging free radical effects which damage cells & might contribute to development of heart disease & cancer. – ods.od.nih.gov

---

Unsaturated oils – preferably cold pressed, are exceptionally rich in vitamin E. Combine oil (olive, safflower, flax) with fresh lemon or orange juice or Bragg Organic Raw Apple Cider Vinegar and Bragg Aminos as healthy dressing for salads. (See recipe page 150)

Organic Non-GMO Whole Grains – Staff of Life

When you buy bread, be sure to select only 100% organic non-GMO whole grain breads. It's fun to bake your own. We try to bake a delicious variety of breads once a week. Try the healthy, delicious (over 700) recipes in the Bragg *Vegetarian Recipe* Book. (See back pages for book list.)

Another good food source of vitamin E and nutrients is cornmeal mush (below) made with organic stoneground yellow cornmeal from health stores (not the refined, degerminated variety found in commercial stores).

Bragg Family's Favorite Cornmeal Recipe

1 Cup organic cornmeal yellow stoneground
3 to 3 1/2 cups distilled water
3 Tbsps raisins, sliced prunes or dates (optional)
1 Tbsp Organic Nut Butter* for topping (optional)

Moisten meal with 2 cups cold water. Boil balance of water, then slowly add moistened cornmeal and raisins. Mix well. When evenly thickened, place in top of double boiler (or put pot in pan of water) with low heat so not to burn! Cook 15 minutes. Serve hot. Top with honey, blackstrap molasses, agape nectar or 100% pure maple syrup (our favorite) and sliced fresh organic fruit (banana, apples, berries, peaches are delicious). Optional toppings: Rice Dream, nut, coconut, soy non-milks, even Nut Butter,

Note: If you are serving this to only a few people, there might be some left over. Put in a flat pan, cool, refrigerate. For breakfast or a main meal, slice and dip in egg (use fertile, free range) batter, and roll in wheat germ flakes. Lightly sauté in soy or olive oil. Serve hot. For variety this cornmeal is delicious topped with poached egg and a little 100% maple syrup or Bragg Blend.

*Organic Nut Butters (almond, peanut, etc.) delicious in oatmeal and hot cereals, stir in cereal just before serving. – PB

Raw wheat germ, besides supplying body with vitamin E, is an important source of organic iron and copper. Other good sources for these minerals are blackberries, blackstrap molasses, dried unsulphured apricots, raw nuts and seeds, dandelion greens, collards, kale, dates, and fertile free-range egg yolks (see page 160).

*For delicious homemade Organic Nut Butters – see page 128.

Vitamin E-Rich Healthy Foods Are Important For Your Health

Here's a list of healthy foods that contain the following notable amounts of precious vitamin E. Buy organic sources – they are best! Reference from National Institute of Health.

Food	Quantity	Vitamin E IU's
Apples	1 medium	1.21
Almonds	1/4 cup	13.37
Bananas	1 medium	0.40
Barley	1/2 cup	4.20
Beans, navy	1/2 cup	3.60
Bell Peppers	1 cup slices	0.94
Blueberries	1 cup	2.18
Broccoli	1 cup	1.12
Butter (salt-free)	6 tablespoons	2.40
Carrots	1 cup	0.45
Celery, green	1/2 cup	2.60
Corn oil	1 tablespoon	2.83
Eggs, fertile	2	2.62
Grapefruit	1/2	0.52
Kale	1/2 cup	8.00
Lettuce	6 leaves	0.50
Olive Oil (virgin)	1 tablespoon	2.38
Onions, raw	2 medium	0.26
Oranges	1 small	0.24
Papaya	1 medium	5.06
Peas, green	1 cup	4.00
Potatoes, white	1 medium	0.06
Potatoes, sweet	1 small	4.00
Rice, brown	1 cup cooked	2.40
Rye	1/2 cup	3.00
Soybean Oil	1 tablespoon	2.24
Sunflower Seeds, raw	1 oz.	8.94
Tomato	1 medium	1.01
Wheat Germ Oil	1 tablespoon	26.20

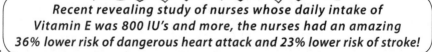

Recent revealing study of nurses whose daily intake of Vitamin E was 800 IU's and more, the nurses had an amazing 36% lower risk of dangerous heart attack and 23% lower risk of stroke!

Wheat Germ – Nature's Health Miracle

My father and I have found this to be true among the athletes we advised. Australian, Murray Rose, youngest Olympic triple gold medal winner in history, who eventually won six Olympic medals in distance swimming – took 400 IUs of vitamin E daily and increased it to 1,500 IUs during competition. Wheat germ, prime source of vitamin E, is also an integral part of the training of most top athletes.

Many decades ago when my health pioneer father first introduced the important need for wheat germ and vitamin E supplements to America, he was called a *faddist*. (Paul C. Bragg gave Viobin it's start, today the world's largest wheat germ company.) It's gratifying that today, in these turbulent health care times, his health teachings have finally been substantiated by worldwide scientific research, both laboratory and clinical, in the fields of biochemistry, exercise, nutrition, water and medicine.

Finally people realized that they rob themselves of the *staff of life – vitamin E* when they make bread from refined white flour (*staff of death*). It's tragic that it took over 80 years and caused millions needless premature deaths and overall health deterioration throughout America and worldwide. White flour has been stripped of its precious wheat germ, nature's best vitamin E source. Everyone who tries to live on the modern civilized diet with refined white flour products devoid of whole grains, suffers from vitamin E deficiency. This has ill effects on people of all ages. Widespread vitamin E deficiency is one of the prime factors in the disastrous increase in heart problems, strokes, heart attacks, cancer and illness!

Scientists at Department of Agriculture's Human Nutrition Research Center on Ageing in Boston report that daily requirements for vitamins B6, B12, C, D and E escalate with age, along with need for calcium, beta carotene and folic acid. Play it safe, also take natural multi-vitamin and mineral supplements.

The USDA has issued new dietary guidelines encouraging us to eat more fresh, organic vegetables and fruits! The guidelines stress the use of dietary sources of vitamins and minerals, especially antioxidants and B vitamins, including folic acid. In addition, diet is important to health at all stages of life and can help reduce the risk of diseases of all kinds.

Locations in the Body Where Osteoporosis, Arthritis, Pain and Misery Hit the Hardest

OUCH!

33 SPINAL VERTEBRAE

RIBS

HUMERUS

HIPS

NECK OF FEMUR

SMALL BONES OF HAND

KNEES

SMALL BONES OF FEET

OSTEOPOROSIS
Affects over 54 Million and Kills over 400,000 Americans Annually

Now an estimated 54 million Americans age 50 or older suffer from osteoarthritis.

Boron: Miracle Trace Mineral For Strong, Healthy Bones

BORON – A trace mineral for healthier bones that also helps the body absorb more vital calcium, minerals and necessary hormones! Good boron sources are most organic veggies, fresh and sun-dried fruits, avocados, prunes, raw nuts and soybeans.

The U.S. Dept. of Agriculture's Nutrition Lab in Grand Forks, ND, says boron is usually found in soil and foods, but many Americans eat a diet low in boron. They conducted a 17 week study which showed a daily 3 to 6 mgs. boron supplement enabled participants to reduce loss (demineralization) of calcium, phosphorus and magnesium from their bodies. This loss is usually caused by eating processed fast foods, drinking tap waters (distilled is best), and eating lots of meat, salt, sugar and fat and a dietary lack of fresh vegetables, fruits and whole grains. (*all-natural.com*)

After 8 weeks on boron, participants' calcium loss was cut 40%. It also helped double important hormone levels vital in maintaining calcium and healthy bones. Millions on estrogen replacement therapy for osteoporosis may want to use boron as a healthier choice.✱ Also consider natural progesterone (2%) raw yam cream. For pain, joint healing use Braggzyme (see page 244) and glucosamine/chondroitin/MSM combo (caps or liquid).

Scientific studies show women benefit from healthy lifestyle that includes vitamin D3 sunshine and exercise (even weight lifting) to maintain healthier bones, combined with purified distilled water, low-fat, high-fiber, carbohydrate, and fresh organic fruits, salads, sprouts, greens and vegetable diet. This healthy lifestyle helps protect against heart disease, high blood pressure, cancer and many other ailments! I'm happy to see science now agrees with my Dad who first stated these health truths in 1920's.

Wrong hard waters cause of most human illness. – Dr. Charles Mayo, Mayo Clinic

✱ *For more hormone and osteoporosis facts read pioneer John Lee, M.D.'s book* – "What Your Doctor May Not Tell You About Menopause" (amazon.com)

Chapter 19

Doctor Rest – The Recharger of Life

Doctor Rest is another health specialist always at your command to help you achieve Supreme Vitality and Health! We believe the word *rest* is the most misunderstood word in the English language. Some people's idea of resting is to sit down and drink a cup of a strong stimulant such as coffee, black tea or caffeinated soft drinks. This is typified by the *coffee break*. To us, rest means repose, freedom from activity and quiet tranquility. It means peace of mind and spirit. It means to rest without anxiety or worry! Rest means to refresh and should renew your whole nervous system and your entire body – physically, mentally, and spiritually.

When you're resting, you shouldn't sit with one leg crossed over the other because this position puts a heavy burden on the popliteal artery which supplies the feet with blood and also cuts off nerve energy. If you sit with legs crossed you are not resting, but giving your heart an extra load of work to do! When you sit down, it's best to keep both feet on the floor or a footstool (see page 175).

To rest means to allow free circulation (no restrictions) of blood throughout the body, which is important for health. Are your shoes too tight? Your collar? Your hat? Your stockings? Your watch, belt, undergarments, bra*****? If yes, then you're not resting when you sit or lie down!

Why do we rest? Often people say, *"I need to rest!"* Yet when they sit down intending to rest, they nervously drum their fingers on a table or desk, quiver or shake their legs or they squirm and move about restlessly (pages 18, 46 and 55).

The art of resting is something that must be acquired and concentrated upon! The best rest can only be secured when your body is relaxed and freed from restrictive clothing! Your clothes should be comfortably loose.

**Read "Dressed To Kill" by S. Singer, on breast cancer & bra studies (amazon.com). Women, please cut wires out of bras that hinder your breast circulation! I've never worn a bra, only a loose chemise. – Patricia Bragg, ND, PhD.*

Enjoy Rest & Naps – It's Not a Crime to Relax!

One good way to rest is to lie down on a firm bed, unclothed or wearing as few, loose clothes as possible. Another way to rest is to sunbathe, see pages 195-198. There is nothing that will relax the muscles and nerves like the gentle, soothing early morning or late afternoon sunrays. In order to rest and nap, you must learn to clear your mind of all anxiety, worries and emotional problems. When the muscles and nerves are relaxed, the heart action slows – especially when you take long, slow, deep breaths! This will help promote a deeper relaxation and more total rest that promotes more total health!

Another good form of resting is a short nap. When you take a nap, command your muscles to become completely relaxed. Your conscious and subconscious mind controls the muscles and the nerves, so you must be in complete command of your body when you rest. Jesus said to His Disciples, when worn and weary, "Come ye and rest a while." The Master did not lead them into the busy streets of Jerusalem where there was noise and clatter. He didn't even take them into the church. He took them into the quiet wide open spaces of nature, under the blue sky. There they could rebuild, relax and revive every organ of their exhausted bodies and also revitalize, refresh and invigorate their weary minds! The greatest place to rest, relax and renew your body's Vital Force is under the blue sky, in the clean, fresh air. On hot summer days, enjoy the cool shade of trees.

Say Good-Bye to Tiredness – Hello Super Energy

- *Sit down and kick off your shoes. Let tiredness go away and now relax!*

- *Now start breathing in easily and deeply, then breathe out tiredness. Next breathe deeply in a feeling of complete peace and relaxation.*

- *Curl your toes down tight, now relax toes and feet. Repeat exercise: Now tighten, then relax fingers and slowly do arms, legs, butt, etc.*

- *Breathe out slowly all the pressures and tiredness of the day. Then breathe in refreshing joy, health, love and peace.*

- *Now relax, close eyes for 10 minutes, then after stand up and stretch.*

- *Stand, stretch arms up, now do wide windmill circles, then reverse circles.*

- *Now stretch your body, arms and legs – sideways, up and down, etc.*

164

Sleep – The Body's Miracle Recharger

Sleep is the greatest revitalizer we have, but few people get a long, peaceful and refreshing night's sleep. Most people habitually use stimulants like tobacco, drugs, coffee, tea and other caffeinated drinks which batter tired nerves! People who use these toxic stimulants never have complete rest and relaxation because nerves are always in an excited condition.

Most people do not earn their rest. Rest must be earned with physical and mental activity, because they go hand in hand. So many people complain what poor sleepers they are – that they toss and turn throughout the night. For an extra relaxer before bedtime try our Bragg Apple Cider Health Drink hot or cold, it's delicious; see recipe on page 149. (More on sleep pages 95-104.)

Sadly millions take some type of drug or alcohol to induce sleep, but this is not true sleep! No one gets restful sleep with sleeping drugs or alcohol. You may drug yourself into unconsciousness, but that very drug will deprive you of a normal, restful, healthy, recharging and satisfying sleep.

Healthy Lifestyle Promotes Sound Sleep

Your nerves are continually irritated when you do not eliminate the toxins from your body. How is it possible to get a good night's rest with irritated nerves? When we faithfully live our Bragg Healthy Lifestyle, exercise, breathe deeply and perform weekly 24 hour fasts, we enjoy and earn sound sleep! We discovered that when our students discard their stimulants and begin a regular fasting program, they too enjoy a more restful, deep sleep.

You will notice as you purify your body that you will be able to relax more readily. You will be able to enjoy naps and you will reap the benefits of a long, restful, night's sleep. Rest is important! The Bible tells us that God appointed one day of rest every week for man. In this wise law, we have ample support for our contention that frequent changes of activity is an important factor in maintaining Super Health. To complement our busy days, we require and enjoy a variety of fun recreational activities. This old adage is true and wise advice to follow: *All work and no play does make Jack and Jill dull and tired.*

Life is to be Savored and Enjoyed – Not Hectic

Today we live in a hectic, competitive environment, which the business world calls the *rat race*. During these stressful times filled with political and emotional unrest, we build up tremendous pressures, tensions and strains. This is why people turn to tobacco, drugs, coffee, alcohol and other harmful substances – to try to escape the stress.

There is not only competition in the business world, but in family and social realm as well, as people strive to maintain their *status*. People are always trying to impress one another and trying to create a certain *image*. Often they create a false image and it takes energy to portray this falseness! There is tremendous pressure on women who believe their worth is being dependent on their appearance. So they spend hours having their hair and nails colored, constantly trying to keep up with the latest fashions, struggling to have a different – *perfect* – body. All of this calls for energy. Our modern civilization drives and pushes us, robbing us of our natural, peaceful state.

It's no wonder we have created millions of alcoholics and drug addicts! Why have people completely forgotten that life is meant to be lived and enjoyed? Too few individuals these days enjoy leisure living. Life is one big rush! Where and why is everyone rushing these days? It's best to slow down, relax – get healthy and be happy!!!

To be able to relax, rest and sleep you must program your day so you have balanced time for work, rest, recreation, exercise and then a good night's sleep. Also, you can't get a good sleep if you overload your stomach! You will enjoy better sleep if you earn it with daily exercise, brisk walking, gardening, etc. We have love and concern for you and love being your health teachers and friends to inspire you to live The Bragg Healthy Lifestyle! Please nourish your body with healthy natural foods, pure distilled water, lots of fresh air, exercise and deep breathing exercises.

Peace is not a season, it's an important way for a healthy life!

I have the wisdom of my years and youthfulness of Bragg Healthy Lifestyle. I never act or feel my calendar years! I feel ageless! So why shouldn't you? Start living this Bragg Healthy Way today! – Dr. Patricia Bragg

Love Mother Nature, God and Yourself Daily

Enjoy a balanced program of exercise and repose and let Mother Nature and God do the rest! Treat yourself as you deserve and the results will astound you! We, the *Back to Nature People*, have been ridiculed for years as faddists and extremists. Now our healthy lifestyle is in demand! The popular press prints stories daily confirming what we have always known! We believe in Mother Nature and God and want to spread their health, joy, peace, happiness and love worldwide. In bible read *3 John 2* and *Genesis 6:3*.

We recommend that you return to a more natural way of living in food, clothing, rest and in simplicity of living habits. Strive for harmony with Mother Nature and God. Live as Mother Nature wants. Realize that she loves you and you are part of her family. Put yourself in her hands and let her inner wisdom guide you. Mother Nature is eager to inspire and guide you so she can help you perfect your human machine. She can help cleanse, heal and improve your body if you work with her by living a healthier life! Please follow the Bragg Healthy Lifestyle.

When possible, leave the smog-filled, air-polluted cities for the country. In the quiet beauty of meadow and hill, you will rekindle your youth. For success: plan, plot and follow through with a strong belief you will become healthier and more youthful! If you live in a city, make it a point to go enjoy your parks, the country, walk the hills, valleys, or the seashore where you can find clean air, relaxation, in a peaceful natural setting for beautiful, recharging retreat time for your body, mind and soul.

Aromatherapy – A Healer For Centuries

Aromatherapy is the practice of using natural oils extracted from flowers, leaves, bark or other parts of a plant to enhance psychological and physical well-being. The inhaled aroma from these "essential" oils is widely believed to stimulate brain function. Essential oils can also be absorbed through the skin, where they travel through the bloodstream and can promote whole-body healing. Aromatherapy has the power to work miracles, to uplift and heal. Treat yourself to the delights and fragrances of essential oils. Smelling beautiful roses, flowers and fruit blossoms is also recharging. See more info on Aromatherapy on page 208. – (AromaTherapy.com)

167

Wise Tips for Healthy, Peaceful Living

● Regard your body as a wonderful miracle machine, 100% under your care and control! Become your own health captain and guardian of your habits of living so you may be well balanced for a long lifetime of health.

● Demand of yourself a higher standard of healthy lifestyle habits! Recognize that every machine must have rest periods! You can't receive higher, super health unless your body gets its rest periods to develop new found vitality and boundless energy! Without sufficient rest, health problems build up when your vital nerve force is depleted. Sadly majority of Americans are stressed-out and unhealthy. Read Bragg *Nerve Force* book (pages 237-239) for more info about building powerful, healthy, peaceful nerves.

● You will become wiser and more mature when you draw closer to and become more intimate with God and Mother Nature! Stop seeking over-stimulation and thrills; instead, seek a simple, "back to nature" peaceful life! Be faithful and you will have a healthy, long and active life God and Mother Nature intended for you to enjoy.

Man's days shall be 120 years. – Genesis 6:3

● With a clear eye and confidence, put yourself in their loving care. They will run your human machine, heal your hurts, comfort you in sickness and adversity. Then, when you have lived a long life of usefulness and happiness, you will be called home (Psalms 23). Make them your life partner, and when you are resting, relaxing, and building new energy, they will always be there for you! So be a child of God and Mother Nature – don't look for sophisticated thrills! Find your fun in nature and diversion in relaxation and other pursuits that are simple as 1, 2, 3. Your rewards will be many: renewed health, calm spirit and a new awareness of the perfect beauties that Mother Nature and our Creator have so generously bestowed on us!

You are encircled by the arms of the mystery of God. – Hildegard of Bingen

---

Just by paying attention to breathing, you can access new levels of health and relaxation that will benefit every area of your life. – Deepak Chopra, M.D.

---

168 *Romance with God and Mother Nature never grows stale, they walk with you and talk with you and their wisdom is thrilling!* – Patricia Bragg, ND, PhD.

Chapter 20

The Importance of Doctor Good Posture

Sit, Stand and Walk Tall for Super Health!

Humans – from head to feet – are built to stand, sit and walk erect. Now that we have reviewed the way your breathing apparatus operates, you can readily understand how correct posture is essential to correct breathing. When you slump, you squeeze your vital organs and lungs into a cramped position that seriously limits the operation of your diaphragm. You become a shallow breather, able to use only the top portion of your lungs. When you sit bent over a desk, you rob your body of maximal oxygen intake, impair circulation, hamper the functions of your heart and vital organs and crowd your muscles and bones into unnatural positions! Then you wonder why you're so fatigued! You probably also cross your legs, which further blocks circulation, preparing the way for broken capillaries, varicose veins, backaches, headaches and a host of unhealthy problems.

It is likely that you maintain the same poor posture when on your feet – standing or walking with your shoulders and head drooping or neck upthrust. You cannot improve matters by suddenly going to the opposite extreme: distorting your body and all of its components by an exaggerated reversal (i.e., thrusting shoulders back and sucking in stomach). You can and will improve and maintain good posture by strengthening your muscles with daily exercise and by daily practicing correct posture habits! *Start now – it works miracles!*

GOOD AND BAD WAYS TO:

Walk   **Sit**   **Lounge**

Right   Wrong   Right   Wrong   Right   Wrong

Learn by doing – Remember practice makes perfect.

*Poor posture can decrease breathing capacity by as much as 30%!
That means there's 30% less oxygen getting to your brain and other cells.*

Posture Can Make or Break Your Health!

Why should emphasis be placed upon such a simple thing as the pull of gravity? In your youth, your muscles held your skeleton in proper balance free from strain or discomfort. Perhaps now circumstances have caused your muscles to lose the battle with gravity. Maybe premature ageing, excess weight or an enforced rest has weakened your muscles just enough to cause your frame to be in an uncomfortable state of balance.

PERFECT POSTURE AND ALIGNMENT

This sagging stretches the ligaments of your back and causes backaches, and when stretched too far they become painful. They are meant to serve only as check reins for the joints and cannot be forcibly stretched without pain. When the ligaments in your back are made uncomfortable by excessive stretching, it is natural for your muscles to try to oppose this gravitational pull. However, if your muscles are too weak to do their proper job, they will rapidly become exhausted and develop the misery of fatigue, making your back painful and uncomfortable.

Check your own symptoms! Do you notice a deep aching and soreness along your spine due to stretched ligaments? Are your back and shoulder muscles achy and tired? Do you have a postural backache caused by weak muscles and bad posture? If so, start now to strengthen your muscles with proper posture and exercise.

Your Health Friend is Doctor Posture

Look at yourself in the mirror! Do your shoulders slump? Is your upper back round? Do you have a potbelly? Are you swaybacked? Can you see the reasons why your back has the right to ache? The bending, slumping, ligament-stretching force of gravity has finally taken charge. Even though you might be a sufferer of backaches due to poor muscles and bad posture, don't despair. With good exercise and good posture habits, plus living The Bragg Healthy Lifestyle you can regain your back and joint comfort!

POSTURES

WRONG RIGHT

WHERE DO YOU STAND?

POSTURE CHART

	PERFECT	FAIR	POOR
HEAD			
SHOULDERS			
SPINE			
HIPS			
ANKLES			
NECK			
UPPER BACK			
TRUNK			
ABDOMEN			
LOWER BACK			

Your posture carries you through life from your head to your feet. This is your human vehicle and you are truly a miracle! Cherish, respect and always protect it by living The Bragg Healthy Lifestyle. – Patricia Bragg

Good posture helps prevent backaches and related problems.

Remember – Your posture can make or break your health!

171

Good Posture – First Step to Healthy Living

Poor posture puts your heart, lungs and all of your *working machinery* into a viselike grip which impairs operations, circulation and efficiency. Keep saying to yourself, *"I must stretch up tall and lift up my chest and diaphragm."* Now, you will be exercising during all of your waking hours. Good posture brings inner strength and tone to your organs and muscles that no exercise can provide.

Correct posture is vital for health and longevity! Keep a straight line from the chin to the toes when standing. Don't slump in your chair when sitting. Keep the head, chest and diaphragm held high. This may tire you at first, but only because your unused muscles are being re-awakened and trained! Once you give strength and tone to the many muscles that control your posture (some also help hold your internal organs), you will find it's easy to maintain good posture. The health rewards are many and you will look and feel healthier and more youthful. To be alive and thrill to the joy of living, you must learn to breathe correctly! Relearning correct posture and breathing habits helps you to attain and maintain the healthy breathing practices you had as a baby. You must learn to breathe with every cell of your lungs. It is then that you can raise your rate of physical vibration to its highest level for healthy super energy.

Normalize Figure with Good Posture & Exercise

You can actually create a more fit body and a normal figure by using correct posture and breathing exercises and living The Bragg Healthy Lifestyle – begin now! All deep breathing exercises are body-building exercises. This is because oxygen is the invisible food – the staff of life, the life-giving miracle force of the body's 75 trillion cells and the vital compliment of the body's assimilation of dietary food. These exercises will help build up a person who is underweight and trim down a person who is overweight. You can burn off fat by internal combustion. You can tone your body and keep it that way. Start now to normalize your figure into its naturally pleasing curves with correct deep breathing habits, along with brisk walking, regular exercise and healthy, wholesome food.

A strong body makes a strong mind. – Thomas Jefferson, 3rd U.S. President (1801–1809)

Bragg Posture Exercise Brings Miracles
Do This Exercise Daily and Practice Good Posture!

Stand tall with feet 9 to 12 inches apart. Tighten your butt and suck in stomach muscles. Lift up rib cage, stretch up spine, hold chest up, shoulders back and lift chin up slightly. Line up your spine – put finger on nose, plumb line straight to belly button, drop arms to sides and swing them to normalize your posture. Look in the mirror to see improvements. Do this posture exercise often; wonderful changes will occur! You are retraining and strengthening your muscles to stand straight for a healthier, fit body with more energy and youthfulness. Stand, walk and sit tall!

Wear Loose, Comfortable Clothing

Don't spoil your health with restrictive clothing such as tight belts, collars, undergarments, bras (page 163) and even tight shoes for they can hamper breathing, blood circulation and the functioning of major organs. It can also throw your body and posture off balance. Today teenagers tend to wear clothes either too loose or too tight!

Which Posture Do You Have?

| GOOD | FAIR | POOR | VERY POOR |

A) GOOD: Head, trunk, thigh in straight line; chest high and forward; abdomen flat; and back curves normal.

B) FAIR: Head forward; abdomen prominent; exaggerated curve in upper back; slightly hollowed back.

C) POOR: Relaxed (fatigued) posture; head forward and down; abdomen relaxed; shoulder blades prominent; hollowed back.

D) VERY POOR: Head forward and down; exaggerated curve in upper back; abdomen relaxed; chest flat-sloping; hollowed back.

How we stand and how we sit affects how we breathe. If the body is slumped over, the shoulders become rounded and the rib cage collapses, giving the lungs no room to expand. Notice the difference in your ability to breathe deeply when you are slumped over a desk or when you are sitting erectly, giving the lungs a chance for maximum expansion.

He who breathes the most air, lives the better life. – Elizabeth Barrett Browning

Learn to Stand, Sit and Walk Tall
For Body Strength and Super Health

To maintain and keep in a healthy state involves many factors including healthy natural food, deep breathing, exercise, rest, sleep, control of emotions and mind, fasting and good posture. If you nourish and give your body loving care, good posture is natural. Conversely, when your body lacks any of these essentials, poor posture is usually the result. Once you have established poor habits, you will have to take definite and corrective measures! You will need to exercise regularly and practice good postural habits in order to restore your natural, healthy stature.

When you sit, your spine should be straight against the chair and both feet should be squarely on floor or foot stool. Your abdominal cavity should be drawn in. Keep shoulders back and hold your chest and head high, never forward. Your arms may be relaxed or lightly clasped in your lap.

When you walk, imagine that your legs are attached to the middle of your chest. This will give you long, gliding, graceful steps. When you walk correctly with this swing and spring, you will naturally build energy. **Your habits either make or break you! Good posture habits help make graceful, strong bodies. Remember this –**

As the twig is bent, so is the tree inclined.

When you sit, keep your torso up and relaxed. Sit squarely on your bottom (it's padded). Keep your feet flat on the floor or with ankles lightly crossed. You can work for hours at your desk in this position without fatigue, but it's best to stop hourly for a good body stretch. Stand, stretch your spine up and do some shoulder rolls forward, then backwards. Then for more energy do some arm-wide swinging windmills (see page 194). Also take frequent brisk walks, maintaining healthy posture with your arms swinging and breathing deeply in rhythm with your stride.

Poor posture can bring unbearable pain across your upper back and fatigue in your drooping shoulders. It can cause weakness in your hips and loins, a numb feeling at your tail bone and often, shooting pain down your legs. Bad posture can develop aches and pains all over the body.

Don't Cross Your Legs – It's Unhealthy

When sitting never cross your legs! Under the knees run two of the largest arteries, called popliteal arteries carrying nourishing blood to the muscles below the knees and to nerves in the feet. You immediately cut down the blood flow to a trickle when you cross your legs.

When the muscles of the legs and knees are not nourished and don't have good circulation, then the extremities stagnate, which can lead to varicose veins or broken and other problems. Look at the ankles of people age 40 and over who have the habit of crossing their legs. Note the broken veins and capillaries. When the muscles and feet do not get their full supply of blood, the feet become weak and poor circulation sets in. Cold feet usually torment the leg-crosser.

DON'T EVER CROSS LEGS!

A well-known heart specialist was asked, "When do most people have a heart attack?" He answered, "At a time they are sitting quietly with one leg crossed over the other." When you sit, plant both feet squarely on the floor or a box if needed. Crossing your legs puts an unnecessary burden on your heart!

People who are habitual leg-crossers have more acid crystals stored in the feet than those who never cross their legs. Crossing the legs is one of the worst postural habits of man. It throws the hips, spine and head off balance and it's the most common cause of chronic backaches, headaches and varicose veins. Be kind to your body – please don't cross your legs. You can break this bad habit.

The Dangers of Sitting too Long

Adjustable Height Desk

Go from sitting to standing easily with the Varidesk. See website: www.VariDesk.com

People who sit too long at work may develop a thrombosis (blood clot) in the deep veins of the calf. If your office work requires you to sit a lot at a computer, *get up, move around every hour* ◀ *or get this desk.*

175

Over 31 Million Americans Suffer Backaches

It has been said that a backache is the penalty people must pay for the privilege of standing and walking upright on two feet. Although some people erroneously believe our ancestors walked on all fours, it's an indisputable fact that we are definitely two-footed. Infants struggle instinctively to stand on their feet and walk! They need not be taught! They attempt a bipedal mode even if left alone most of the time and never instructed. It's absolutely natural for human beings to stand and walk in this manner. This is especially interesting in light of the fact that no other animals spend all of their standing and walking hours on two feet, not even the primates that are most like us – chimpanzees and apes. Human beings are designed to walk upright and animals are not!

The spines of humans have normal curves that enable muscles to oppose gravity and hold the back erect. As long as the muscles are strong enough to maintain balance and prevent a sagging camel-back, the back is comfortable. When muscles are too weak to work, the back sags, ligaments are stretched and then the inevitable happens – a backache, that sadly affects millions of Americans!

Good posture is an important part of breathing. For correct posture, align your body with an imaginary vertical line from the top center of your head through the center of your pelvis to the floor between your feet. Do the Bragg Posture Exercises page 65-66, 173 often. For more back exercises, etc. read the Bragg *Back Fitness Program* book, pages 237-239.

Now establish this simple, incredibly beneficial habit: stand tall, walk tall and sit tall. When this healthy posture becomes a habit, the result is correct posture! Any sagging, prolapsed vital organs will slowly assume and take their normal positions and function better. Daily faithfully follow The Bragg Healthy Lifestyle and drink 8 glasses of pure distilled water and always practice good posture.

Poor posture inhibits the flow of oxygen throughout the body. With less oxygen taken in, every cell in the body then becomes undernourished and hungry for fresh oxygen. Of paramount importance is the circulation to the head area. Because of gravity, blood carrying oxygen naturally has to work harder to get up above the heart into the head. When poor posture interferes with circulation it also affects skin, eyes, organs, brain, hair. – Philip Smith, "Total Breathing" (amazon.com)

Your back and your feet carry you through life – be good to them!

Chapter 21

Doctor Fresh Air

Dr. Fresh Air is a Super Health Specialist and his greatest health prescription for a long, healthy, fulfilled life is . . .

> ### *The Breath of God's Pure Fresh Air,*
> ### *Is The Invisible Staff of Life.*

The first thing we do when we are born is to take a long, deep breath and the final thing we do is take a last gasp before we stop breathing. Between birth and death our whole life is completely maintained by our breathing!

Dr. Fresh Air wants you to have a long, healthy life. Practice these Bragg Super Power Breathing Exercises and remain conscious that with every breath you take you are bringing into your body precious life-giving oxygen! People who fail to obey the doctor's orders about getting plenty of fresh air day and night invite many severe complications. Let us examine the function of breathing. Air is invisible food – the only food that we absolutely cannot live without! If we are deprived of air for over 5 to 7 minutes, death takes us! **We are miracle breathing machines! Nurture, protect and honor your precious life!**

Air supplies us with life-giving oxygen CO_2, which is critical for every cell in our bodies. Oxygen is carried by the blood to the lungs where miracles takes place: the exchange of life-giving oxygen for deadly carbon dioxide. We create deadly toxins in the process of living that CO_2 carries out of our bodies. These are collected by our blood, brought to our lungs and expelled as the new life-giving oxygen enters our bloodstream! During the process of metabolism, the building up and tearing down of the cells of the body, and in the very process of living, carbon dioxide poison is constantly burned up and expelled.

You are what you breathe, eat, drink, think, say & do!
– Patricia Bragg, ND, PhD., Pioneer Health Crusader

Our breathing is a miracle process to support the ongoing miracle awareness of life in running our daily lives. – Jon Kabat-Zinn, PhD.

Man's days shall be to 120 years. – Genesis 6:3

We are Miracle Air Breathing Machines

When a person does not get enough fresh air – or is a shallow breather – and their intake of oxygen does not equal the output of carbon dioxide, then this poison can build up in the body. This could result in serious physical problems because the retained carbon dioxide can be concentrated in other parts of the body and could cause intense physical problems and body suffering.

Enervation is the lack of nerve energy that lowers the Vital Force so much that the lungs cannot pump in enough air to flush carbon dioxide out of the body. Now you see how important it is to breathe fresh air deeply and be faithful with Super Power Breathing exercises every day!

We are air-pressure machines and oxygen purifies our bodies. It's one of the greatest detoxifiers of the human body. We live at the bottom of an atmospheric ocean approximately 70 miles deep. This air pressure is 14 pounds per square inch. Between the inhalation and the exhalation of a breath, a vacuum is formed. As long as we continue to have this rhythmical intake of oxygen and outflow of carbon dioxide, we will live. We know that we can go without food for 30 days or more and still survive, but we can only go without air for a few minutes. Air is one of the most important energizers of the human body. **The more deeply you breathe, the better your chances for extending your years for a long healthy life on Earth.**

For over 70 years, my father researched long-lived people and found one common factor among them: they are deep breathers! The deeper – and therefore fewer – breaths a person takes in one minute, the longer that person lives. Rapid breathers are short-lived. This holds true in the animal world, too. Rabbits, guinea pigs and all kinds of rodents are rapid breathers, taking many breaths every minute. They are among the shortest-lived creatures on the face of Earth. For years we have made it a practice to take long, slow, deep breaths when we first get up in the morning. During the day, we also try to take 3-5 minute breaks where we breathe long, deeper full breaths. Try this now – it makes you feel wonderfully alive!

Indian Holy Men Practice Slow, Deep Breathing and Prayer Meditation

On my father's expeditions into India, he found holy men in secluded retreats who devoted their lives to building physically powerful bodies as instruments for high spiritual advancement. They spent many hours daily in the practice of rhythmic, relaxed, long, slow, deep breathing. These holy men of India were utterly fantastic physically. The deep breathing of fresh air kept their skin and muscle-tone ageless. Dad met a holy man in the foothills of the Himalaya Mountains who told him that he was 126 years old. This man's whole life was spent getting closer to God, and he is the one who taught my father the system which we expanded upon and now teach around the world . . . *The Bragg Super Power Breathing.*

This holy man had perfect vision and he had a beautiful head of hair. He had all his teeth and the endurance and stamina of an athlete. He also spoke five languages fluently. He was one of the most amazing men my father has ever met! When asked to what he owed his great strength, youthfulness and mentality, he answered, ***"I have made a lifelong practice of faithfully doing my slow, deep breathing and some prayer meditations daily."***

My father does not like to guess the age of any person, but while he was on this trip to India he met a woman whose age he guessed to be about 50. He was amazed when she told him she was 86. She was a beautiful woman with vitality and no sign of age deterioration! He was impressed and asked her the secret of her natural beauty and her agelessness! Again he got the same answer he did from the holy man, this beautiful woman was conscious of the importance of deep, slow breathing and prayer!

"I am not perfect. My mind wanders during my mediation practice and I sometimes feel the difficulties of life get under my skin. I know I need improvement. Happiness and well-being is a process. We make a choice about whether to try to be happy or not. Choosing happiness means cultivating your compassion, your generosity, your concern for others and continuously trying to push any negative thoughts out! The act of cultivating happiness, in and of itself, leads you to more happiness. Keep working on it!" – The Dalai Lama

Super Power Deep Breathing: Secret of Endurance, Stamina & Longevity

How well your lungs function, may predict how long you live. No doubt you have noticed rosy-cheeked children playing – running, jumping rope, skating and bicycling. They inhale large amounts of oxygen while doing these activities, and this we must keep in mind. We must keep active! We must exercise and take long, brisk walks and cultivate deep breathing. When people live sedentary lives and no longer get vigorous exercise, they are harming themselves and shortening their lives. *FraminghamHeartStudy.org* studies showed importance of lifestyle in health and longevity is how well you breathe.

We had a long-time friend named Amos Stagg who was a famous California football and athletic coach. He lived over 100 active, healthy years! We asked him his secret of long life at his 100th birthday party. His answer was, *"I have the greater part of my life indulged in running and vigorous exercise that forced large amounts of oxygen into my body and along with working with athletes, has kept me youthful and interested in staying healthy, fit and alive!"*

Dad had a friend in New York, James Hocking, who was one of the greatest long-distance walking champions this country has ever had. We asked him on his 100th birthday the secret of his long, active, super healthy life. His answer, *"I have always walked vigorously and breathed deeply."* Oxygen is a cleansing detoxifier like fasting. His daily deep breathing helped cleanse the toxins from his body.

Dad and I practice deep breathing and believe people should expose their bodies to free currents of moving air. Air baths are important for good health! Whenever possible do sleep with your windows wide open with cross ventilated air moving across your body. We sleep better and have a deeper night's rest if we wear light sleeping garments of cotton or silk – or nothing at all. You will be warm under the covers. But if you sleep with heavy blankets and nightwear, you smother your skin's vital oxygen supply and increase your chance of illness.

Control your emotions by learning to calmly breathe deeply through them.

Healthy Walking Helps Solve Problems

You will find you can solve most problems on a brisk one to three mile walk. Whenever we have a problem to solve, we take a long brisk walk in the fresh air and even if raining (Bragg follower Conrad Hilton walked rain or shine). By the time we finish our walk, we usually find a solution! We believe everyone should enjoy taking brisk short walks (arms swinging) hour after their evening meal – even if it is up and down their driveway. Today people have become sitters. They sit at their work, movies, concerts, sport events, T.V., web, and computers at home. They are starved for more oxygen, exercise and circulation!

You must compensate for the hours you spend sitting down, because it inhibits your circulation and natural, healthy breathing! If your work and lifestyle require a lot of sitting, you should compensate for it with outdoor brisk walking and more vigorous physical activities daily. When you cannot get the carbon dioxide out of your body, you develop aches, pains and become prone to premature ageing! This is due to lack of physical activity and sufficient oxygen. On city streets, you can see pale, ghostly people, unhealthy and exhausted – mostly as a result of oxygen-starvation and poor lifestyle choices!

It's critical to fast, because it enables you to clean out some of this concentrated, stored-up carbon dioxide that failed to leave your body by deep breathing. When you are fasting, enjoy walking – even if it is a short walk. Make it a regular part of your life to be an active person! This doesn't mean house walks. It means getting out in the fresh air and do brisk walks, hiking, biking, running, tennis, swimming or dancing, etc. You must not allow any carbon dioxide to build up in your body – it will bring you health problems!

Make it a point every day of your life to breathe deeply during a vigorous brisk walk or some other aerobic exercise. Take long, slow, deep breaths every time you think of it. Soon your slow, deep breathing becomes a normal habit. When you combine deep breathing with fasting and living The Bragg Healthy Lifestyle, you are building more health, energy and vitality and you will live longer. Remind yourself daily *Doctor Fresh Air is your very important constant friend!*

HEALTHY HEART HABITS FOR LONG, VITAL LIFE

Remember, organic live foods make live people. *You are what you eat, drink, breathe, think, say and do.* So eat a low-fat, low-sugar, high-fiber diet of organic fresh raw salads, sprouts, greens, vegetables, whole grains, fruits, raw seeds, nuts, fresh juices and chemical-free, purified or distilled water.

Earn your food with daily exercise, for regular exercise, brisk walking, etc. improves your health, stamina, go-power, flexibility, endurance and helps open the cardiovascular system. Only 45 minutes a day truly can do miracles for your heart, arteries, mind, nerves, soul and body! You become revitalized with new zest for living to accomplish your life goals!

We are made of tubes. To help keep them open, clean and to maintain good elimination, take 1 veg psyllium cap or add 1 tsp psyllium husk powder daily – hour after dinner to juices, herbal teas, even Bragg Vinegar Drink. Another way to guard against clogged tubes daily is to add 1-2 tsps soy lecithin granules (*fat emulsifier-melts like butter*) over potatoes, veggies, soups and juices, etc. Also take one cayenne capsule (40,000 HU) daily with a meal. Take 50 to 100 mgs. regular-released niacin (B3) with one meal daily to help cleanse and open the cardiovascular system, also improves memory. Skin flushing may occur, don't worry about this as it shows it's working! After cholesterol level reaches 180, then only take niacin twice weekly.

The heart needs healthy balanced nutrients, so take natural multi-vitamin-mineral food supplements, Omega-3 and extra heart helpers – vitamin E with mixed Tocotrienols, vitamin C, Ubiquinol CoQ10, D3, MSM, D-Ribose, garlic, turmeric, selenium, zinc, beta carotene and amino acids: L-Carnitine, L-Taurine, L-Lysine and Proline. Folic acid, CoQ10, B6 and B12 helps keep homocysteine level low. Magnesium Orotate, Hawthorn Berry Extract helps bring relief for palpitations, arrhythmia, senile hearts and coronary disease. Braggzyme contains systemic enzymes (nattokinase & serrapetase) to help keep blood thin, preventing dangerous blood clots. Take multi-digestive enzyme and probiotics with meals – aids in digestion, assimilation and elimination.

For sleep problems try 5-HTP Tryptophan (an amino acid), melatonin, calcium, magnesium, valerian (in caps, extract or tea), Bragg Vinegar Drink and Sleepytime herb tea. For arthritis or joint pain/stiffness, try aloe juice or gel, Braggzyme, Glucosamine-Chondroitin-MSM combo caps and shots, helps heal and regenerate. Capsaicin and DMSO lotion helps relieve pain. Natural liver cleanses to repair and regenerate include milk thistle, dandelion root, artichoke and turmeric. Dandelion root is a natural diuretic and helps clear toxins through urination and also helps stimulate liver bile flow so waste can be eliminated.

Use amazing antioxidants – E Tocotrienols, Vit C, Quercetin, grape seed extract (OPCs), CoQ10, selenium, SOD, Resveratrol, Alpha-Lipoic Acid, etc. They improve immune system and help flush out dangerous free radicals that cause havoc with cardiovascular pipes and health. Research shows antioxidants promote longevity, slows ageing, fights toxins, helps prevent disease, cancer, cataracts, jet lag and exhaustion.

Recommended Heart Health Tests

- **Total Cholesterol:** Adults: 180 mg/dl is optimal; **Children:** 140 mg/dl or less
- **LDL Cholesterol:** 100 mg/dl or less is optimal
- **HDL Cholesterol:** Men: 50 mg/dl or more; **Women:** 65 mg/dl or more
- **Triglycerides:** 100 mg/dl or less (optimal 70-85)
- **HDL/Cholesterol Ratio:** 3.2 or less • **Triglycerides/HDL Ratio:** below 2
- **Homocysteine:** 6-8 micromoles/L
- **CRP (C-Reactive Protein high sensitivity):**
    lower than 1 mg/L low risk, 1-3 mg/L average risk, over 3 mg/L high risk
- **Diabetic Risk Tests:** • **Glucose:** 80-100 mg/dl • **Hemoglobin A1c:** 7% or less
- **Blood Pressure:** 120/70 mmHg is considered optimal for adults

Chapter 22

Doctor Exercise

Activity is Life, Stagnation is Death

Doctor Exercise makes this assertion . . . *To be lazy is to rust and rust means decay and destruction!* If we don't use our muscles, they loose their tone and life! To keep muscles firm, strong and youthful, they must be continually used! **Activity is the Law of Health and Life! Action is the Law of Well-Being!** All the body's vital organs have specific functions that depend upon health and strength. Regular exercise helps to maintain and normalize weight, blood pressure, blood sugar and your cholesterol and fat levels.

When we exercise, we increase our physical strength, stamina, suppleness and good circulation! Daily exercise improves digestion, elimination and strengthens the muscles, especially the heart! If we are lazy and don't use our 640 muscles, our circulation, muscles and health all suffer from lack of exercise! The unused muscles become flabby, weak, unhealthy and unable to enjoy active exercise and a normal healthy, vigorous, long life.

Regular Exercise Promotes Healthy Skin & Body

People who exercise regularly are happier and have healthier, firmer skin tone. When we exercise, we bring on healthy perspiration from our body's 96 million pores. (Health Clubs have steam and sauna rooms we enjoy that open your pores.) Skin is the body's largest eliminative organ (often called your third kidney). If someone gilded your body, clogging all your pores, you would die within minutes.

When you are exercising and perspiring freely, impurities and toxic poisons are being expelled. This allows the skin to perform its natural function of eliminating these poisons. If you don't exercise daily to the point of some perspiration, the cleansing work that the pores should be doing can throw a burden on the other eliminative organs and then some physical troubles could occur.

If you don't use it, you lose it – it's also true for the mind, body and spirit.

Enjoy Heart Healthy Exercise

Vigorous exercise helps to normalize blood pressure and helps create a healthier pulse. Vigorous exercise acts as an anticoagulant, which means it helps keep the blood from forming the clots which can cause a heart attack or stroke. **Daily exercise and brisk walking works miracles!**

Exercise Promotes Healthy Elimination

Every creature and human eliminates internal waste by means of muscular action. Inside your intestinal tract, there are three muscular layers which undergo a precise rhythmic, *wavelike-squeeze-push* called peristalsis. If you allow the internal and external abdominal muscles (important for elimination) to become inactive, flabby and fat instead of muscular, they lose their power to contract normally. The results: intestinal clogging which can cause constipation and even some diarrhea at times.

What happens when stomach muscles become weak and infiltrated with fat? They often refuse to work regularly. Then intestinal waste that should have been eliminated piles up. Fecal and toxic waste build-ups cause ill health. This sluggish inactivity can cause many serious diseases.

The Importance of Abdominal Exercises

The most important exercises stimulate all muscles of the human trunk from hips to armpits. These are the binding muscles which hold all vital organs in place. In developing your torso muscles, you are also developing vital muscles. As your back, waist, chest and abdomen increase in soundness and elasticity, so will your lungs, liver, heart, stomach and kidneys gain in efficiency and productivity. When exercising regularly, the arch of your ribs widens. This gives free play to lungs. Your elastic diaphragm allows heart to pump and function more powerfully. Your rubberlike waist, in its limber action, stimulates kidneys and massages liver. Your abdominal muscles strengthen and support your stomach with controlled undulations. All this trunk exercise acts like a massage of vital organs and exerts an influence over the whole organism that must not be underestimated – it's so vital for Super Health!

Our best preparation for tomorrow is the wise, proper use of today!

Exercise Relieves Varicose Veins, Ankle and Leg Swelling

If you sit or stand for a long time and your ankles become swollen, lie flat on your back, raise your legs and stretch your feet toward the ceiling and breathe deeply. It also helps to circulate any stagnant pooled blood (varicose veins) by using your hands to gently press downwards from ankles to hips. You will feel the blood flowing from your feet and ankles toward your heart. If you are in a place where you can't do this, breathe deeply in and out while you alternately rise up on your toes, then down and roll up on heels. Deep breathing and muscular action will stimulate circulation and help relieve the venous blood congestion and provide relief for aching legs and feet. These are good exercises upon awakening and before bedtime.

Enjoy Brisk Walks for Healthy Long Life

We recommend most all forms of exercise, but feel daily brisk walking with arms swinging, is the best all-around exercise! This walking moves most of the body. Grasp the small of your back as you walk and feel how your entire frame responds to every stride and how the muscles work rhythmically. Walking promotes harmony of all the body's coordinating muscles. Your daily walk promotes healthier blood circulation, elimination, deeper breathing and helps normalize blood pressure, even diabetes and cholesterol.

Of all the many forms of exercise, brisk walking is the one that brings most of the body into action! It's the *king of exercise* and when the rhythm of your deep breathing and rhythm of your stride are in harmony, you feel more vibrant and alive! As the oxygen-filled blood courses through your body, your legs will carry you along buoyantly. Walk tall with your head held high, back straight, chest up, tummy in, arms swinging easily from your shoulders; legs moving as smoothly as though they were attached to the middle of your torso.

Exercise is a normal state for the body and most people with breathing problems can exercise safely. – Neil F. Gordon, author, "Breathing Disorders" – amazon.com

Brisk Walking is the King of Exercise

Walk briskly at least one to three miles every day and more when you have time. Don't make excuses! Make your daily walk a fixed routine no matter what kind of weather. In stormy weather, walk inside your home, on your porch or driveway, in the mall, etc. When traveling, use hotel hallways, stairs or even the treadmill or exercise equipment in the hotel's gym. **Walking can be done anytime, anywhere. Start today!**

Dad and I always prefer outdoor fresh air walking, but walking indoors is far better than no walking at all. When traveling the world on our Bragg Health Crusade tours, we often take a light jog or a brisk evening walk through the corridors of our hotel or up and down the hotel stairs. Our favorite places for brisk walks are beaches, parks, hills and the open decks of cruise ships for the clean, fresh air.

Walking does not need to be done consciously. No heel and toe business. No getting there within a certain time limit. Let walking be as it is: the most functional of exercises. Carry yourself well. Walk naturally with your head high and chest up! You will feel physically elated and you will carry yourself proudly, straight and erect – yet relaxed and with an easy, smooth arm-swing. Vow to become a wonderful walker and make the day's walk a fixed item in your health program all the year round and in any kind of weather. Go at your own pace with your spirit free. If the outer world of Mother Nature fails to interest you, turn to the inner world of the mind. (Science now says adults can grow new brain cells, see web: *salk.edu*)

In our opinion walking is better than golf. Life has so much to teach us that it's a time-waster trying to get a ball into a hole in a stroke less than another person. Unfortunately most golfers now use electric golf carts which eliminates the best part of golf – walking!

Walking Posture
Always prepare a new foot base before leaving the old one.

Miracle–Walking Builds New Blood Vessels

American Health reported that Dr. Gary Giangola, a vascular surgeon at New York University Medical Center, prescribed walking instead of bypass surgery for one of his patient's atherosclerosis. It was so pervasive it had severely restricted the blood flow to the legs and was causing extreme pain and numbness in his patient's feet. Dr. Giangola told his patient that if he walked one mile every day (even if he had to stop every two blocks to rest and recover), it would help build new blood vessels (collaterals) which would help bypass his closed arteries. He enjoyed his recovery! One year later the patient was able to enjoy walking several miles every day. Start walking!

Organic Gardening is Fun – Plus Exercise

Gardening is a marvelous form of exercise. It gives you exercise in the open air to help keep you more flexible. But you can gain weight even if you garden because there is too little movement. We love walking. Achieve your goals by applying your energy productively in your organic vegetable and flower gardens, then take the kink out of your back with a healthy brisk walk and stretching! Personally, we enjoy combining these: swimming, tennis, biking, calisthenics, hiking and brisk walking. We also love garden exercise. We have a variety of organic fruit trees, vegetables, herbs and flower gardens with over 600 roses. My father said, *"Roses are God's Autograph of Fragrance, Beauty & Love."* *Please visit our rose gardens at Bragg.com*

> *"There is but one way to live and that is Mother Nature's and God's Healthy Way!"*

As a single footstep will not make a path on the earth, so a single thought will not make a pathway in the mind. To make a deep physical path, we walk again and again! To make a deep mental path, we must think over and over the kind of wise thoughts we wish to dominate our lives. – Henry D. Thoreau

---

Make fitness a lifestyle with Flex™ Heart Monitor – WIRELESS ACTIVITY and SLEEP WRISTBAND. This slim wristband device you wear as often as you want, keeps track of your walking distance and even calories burned. If worn at night, it tracks sleep quality and wakes you silently in morning. It's the motivation you need to get walking and be more active!
– fitbit.com • *"I love my pink FitBit – it's a lot of fun, get one!"* – Dr. Patricia

Cold Water Swimmers are Fit and Ageless

My father prides himself on being able to endure the coldest weather wearing only a small amount of clothing, and he has enjoyed swimming in all parts of the world, in all kinds of weather, (which I also enjoy). He is well known for his cold water swimming and is welcomed as a member at Polar Bear Clubs worldwide. On many occasions, Dad and famous pioneer Dr. Robert Jackson

Cold Water Swimmers "L" Street Beach, Boston
Dr. Paul C. Bragg and Dr. John H. Federkiewicz, David Cooper and Dr. David Carmos (the youngest)

had great sport breaking the ice and swimming with the amazing Boston Brownies of the famous "L" Street Bath House in Massachusetts. Here you'll find some of the finest ageless physical specimens in the world, including people in their 60's, 70's, 80's 90's, and even over 100 years.

The same is true of the Polar Bears of Coney Island and at Montrose Beach in Chicago and those at the popular Bradford Beach in Milwaukee, Wisconsin. They are all fit, amazing and ageless. These healthy, hearty people who enjoy swimming in ice-cold water are all deep, full breathers. Many of them follow our Bragg System of Super Power Breathing. When you Super Power Breathe, you enjoy cold water swimming because both deep breathing and swimming are very invigorating and energizing!

We certainly don't recommend that everyone jump into ice-cold water! Let's leave that to people who have developed bodies with perfect thermostatic control. You can start slowly with alternating cold and warm showers. These swimmers are just examples of the power your body can develop when you are filled with oxygen at all times. There is no limit to your powers of resistance or your feeling of well-being when every cell in your body is filled with precious life-giving oxygen!

Studies show that athletes tend to have higher HDL (good cholesterol) levels.

Opera and Broadway Singers, Ballet Dancers and Champion Athletes are Deep Breathers

Breath control, by deep diaphragmatic breathing, is vital for all professional singers. Without benefit of loudspeakers, the voices of the early great opera singers filled the auditoriums of the Metropolitan, La Scala and other famous opera houses throughout the world. What diaphragms they had! Look at the builds of these men and women. They have beautiful, perfect posture; superior development of the torso and tremendous lung capacity. Listen to the great recorded classic voices of Enrico Caruso and Mario Lanza, and those of other tenors who thrilled the world, such as Luciano Pavoratti, Placido Domingo and Jose Carreras. Hear their perfect voice control, from the softest pure note to the swell of a great crescendo. Study the lives of these extraordinary people and you will find that, regardless of their age, their attention to health and deep breathing filled them with energy and charm. Most of these deep breathers live remarkably long, productive, happy lives.

Secret of Hollywood's Dancing Greats: Diaphragmatic Breathing

The same is true of all great dancers. Dad's friends, famous Ruth St. Dennis and Ted Shawn, thrilled audiences throughout their long lifetimes, from their teens into their 70's. Deep diaphragmatic breathing was the key to tremendous energy and muscular control they brought to their spectacular dances! It was also the main key to their long, healthy, vibrant lives filled with super energy.

Deep diaphragmatic breathing is a basic component of the rigorous training of all the famous ballet companies. Many of Hollywood's great dancers like Fred Astaire, Gene Kelly, Arthur Murray and rollicking Rockettes of New York's Radio City Music Hall were living The Bragg Healthy Lifestyle. In order to have super energy, dancers find it's important to live a healthy lifestyle. As a result, most live long lives, maintaining perpetual youthfulness. (P.S. *I've danced with Fred Astaire, Gene Kelly, Lawrence Welk and Arthur Murray – dancing helps keep you young!* – Patricia)

189

The beauty, strength, energy and endurance of North African dancers also amazes me. Their secret is the excellent development of diaphragm breathing. Because their lungs draw in and expel large quantities of fresh air, these women have exquisite skin tone and flawless complexions, sparkling eyes, remarkably graceful and supple bodies.

Even if you aren't a singer or dancer, there is no reason why you shouldn't also enjoy good health and a long, happy, productive life. Without having to undergo the rigorous training of a professional performer, you can profit from their key secrets: deep diaphragmatic breathing, regular exercise, a healthy lifestyle and a natural diet.

Should We Exercise During Fasting?

Only the faster can answer this question. If there is no inclination for physical activity during a fast, then don't exercise. At most do some relaxing stretches and deep breathing! The fast is giving you a physiological rest. Unless you have a big urge for physical activity, you should relax and rest as much as possible when fasting.

During a fast, your body is using all of its Vital Force for internal purification. But if during a 7 to 10 day fast you feel the need for some stretching or walking, respond to the urge. It's between fasts and in your daily program of living that you should spend a portion of every day of your life exercising, preferably outdoors. Soon you will enjoy a more vigorous circulation instead of sluggish one. Poor body circulation causes many health problems, discomfort, pain and misery also throughout the body.

Fasting & Exercise Promotes Health & Energy

Fasting and a healthy lifestyle are your friends in your pursuit of youthfulness, health and symmetry. When it comes to fighting fat – diet and fasting come first! When it comes to keeping fit, exercise matters most. They all help each other; by enjoying daily exercise you may be more generous with your diet and your body machine should work better and enjoy more super efficiency! All machines improve with wise, intelligent use.

Fasting is cleansing, purifying and restful. – Meir Schneider, founder of School for Self-Healing, San Francisco & Author of "Miracle Eyesight Method"

Nothing betrays its weak areas as much as inactivity, and lack of regular maintenance and the inadequate, low-energy fuel! For example: your car needs routine maintenance, including gas, oil changes, tune-ups, etc.

The more you fast, the more toxins you cleanse from your body! As your body increases its internal cleanliness, your muscles will enjoy more energy, tone and vitality. You will find that your old, sluggish, lazy feelings will leave you and then you will desire more action and more physical activity! Life will become more exciting! When people don't exercise, their ankles and legs often swell because there's not enough blood circulating to remove the waste from the cells and carry it back to the organs of elimination! Allow no excuses for not exercising! Regardless of your physical condition, it's vitally important that some form of exercise become a part of your Bragg Healthy Lifestyle! Plot out a plan and get started now!

Exercise Helps avert Sickness and Ageing!

Exercise helps builds a health fund of endurance and resistance! It helps build a healthy bloodstream with balanced white and red corpuscles that help keep us healthy by keeping our immune system on constant guard to fight off any germs, illnesses, etc. Exercise helps maintain a serene and tranquil mind and increases confidence. A 1 to 3 mile brisk walk in the fresh air with God and Mother Nature helps neutralize most all unhealthful emotional upsets! The knowledge that you have improved your mental and physical abilities through exercise will give you supreme confidence. Exercise helps cultivate willpower and gives you control of your Physical, Mental and Spiritual Self which helps you to further promote your personal efficiency, happiness and longevity!

Exercise is the greatest health tonic we can provide ourselves! To attain this feeling of radiant, glorious health, follow The Bragg Healthy Lifestyle and engage in regular, vigorous physical activity. You will look and feel better and more youthful! **Bragg Healthy Lifestyle helps produce miraculous feelings of super, joyous agelessness!**

Regular exercise is a critical part of staying healthy. There are 1,440 minutes in every day. Schedule 30 of them for physical activity! – nlm.nih.gov/hinfo.html

Exercise, deep breathing, healthy foods, with some fasting helps maintain a healthier physical balance for a longer, happier life!

Stop Procrastinating – Start Exercising Daily

When it comes to these exercises – and in fact all exercises and all habits of wise, healthy living – what is truly important is the DOING. "Knowing" and "wanting" are important too. But the "doing" is what it's all about. Don't play counter-productive games with yourself. The moment you begin asking yourself, "Do I have time to do this right now?" is the very moment to stop asking and start doing! The moment you begin to think, "I don't have the energy right now," is the very moment to stop thinking negatively and start doing. Be positive, start now, please no more procrastinating!

Start the 10 Minute Trick – It Works Miracles

The successful student of The Bragg Healthy Lifestyle, and anyone who has successfully made healthy exercise part of their daily routine, will tell you the same thing: The moment of beginning is the most difficult. The in-between moment after you decide you want to become healthier and before you begin to act on that decision is the hardest moment. The moment before you put that one leg in front of the other on the first step of your brisk walk is the most difficult moment of the exercise.

The people who tell the success stories of exercise recommend "tricking yourself" into exercising at first. Play the "10 minute trick". Before you start (the hardest moment), tell yourself, "I'll only exercise, walk, etc. for 10 minutes and then I'll stop. That will be easy and I'll be done soon." Once you've done this, you're on the path to healthy fitness – and it will be fun! Once this most difficult moment is over (the beginning) you'll find when the 10 minute mark comes around that you are enjoying yourself too much to quit so soon!

It's Never Too Late to Start Exercising

Studies show it's never too late to begin exercising. Recent physical activity has a greater positive impact on cardiovascular disease and mortality than exercise done in one's past. The cardiovascular health benefits of recent physical activity are more pronounced than with distant physical activity, even though both are beneficial. A consistent maintenance exercise program produced the best overall results! – Sports Medicine Digest, www.TheSportDigest.com

Progress is impossible without change, and those who cannot change their minds, cannot change anything. – George Bernard Shaw

The journey of a thousand miles begins with one step. – Lao Tzu

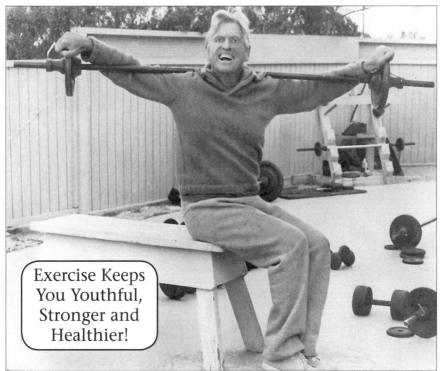

> Exercise Keeps You Youthful, Stronger and Healthier!

Paul C. Bragg and Patricia Lift Weights 3 Times Weekly

Building Up a Healthy Body with Exercise

Exercise helps to normalize blood pressure and create a healthy pulse. It keeps the blood flowing smoothly and not clot. Staying active keeps you feeling energized!

Dr. Fiatarone's Boston study and others have proven that weight-lifting rejuvenates oldsters. They turned a group of frail Boston nursing home residents into weight-lifters to demonstrate it's never too late to reverse age-related decline in muscle strength. This study shows the great importance of keeping the 640 muscles as active and fit as possible to maintain general overall good health! Try it – it works for us and others! Studies conclude: "A 3 days-a-week weight-training program is capable of inducing dramatic increase in health, longevity and muscle strength in frail men and women even up to 96 years of age." See web: *AntiAgingResearch.com/behavioral_factors.shtml* for more info.

Staying active is like riding an UP elevator. The more you do, the more you feel like staying involved. Even couch potatoes can become active and fit!

If exercise could be packed into a pill, it would be the single most widely prescribed and beneficial medicine in America. – Robert Butler, MD

Do These Exercises Daily (10 per set):

You must exercise! It's important because weak muscles of the arms, legs and entire body indicates a similar unhealthy condition also of the stomach muscles and heart (a muscle) and other vital important body organs.

Important Exercises for Keeping External and Internal Muscles of The Stomach and Back Fit and Healthy. These Also Promote Good Elimination and Energy.

Bend at the waist to the sides, then front and back.

Do bicycles and leg kicks.

Do leg and buttock stretches.

Do waist twists and Bragg windmills.

Bragg Windmill Exercise: *Swing arms forward and go around in large circles. Let your hands feel heavy and let the hands carry your arms around and around. Now do backward circles. Breathe easily and deeply, feet 12 inches apart, bend knees a little and then straighten them up with each circle. Do 3 to 5 times daily. Results: tension goes, energy increases!*

Chapter 23

Doctor Gentle Sunshine

Doctor Sunshine's specialty is heliotherapy and his great prescription is solar energy! Each blade of grass, every vine, tree, bush, flower, fruit and vegetable draws its life from solar energy. All living things on earth depend on solar energy for their existence. The earth would be a barren, frigid place if it were not for the magic sun rays! The sun gives us light, and were it not for light, there would be no you or me! Earth would be in total darkness and void of life. (We use and endorse solar energy when and where possible.)

A person's skin is gently tanned by the sun and air and will take on a darker pigment according to its original type. It has been found that with gentle exposure to the sun even redheaded people will eventually tan. Pigmentation is a sign that solar energy has been transformed into human energy. Mankind can gain health, vitality and happiness in gentle, healing rays of the sun (page 197).

The people who are indoors too long have sallow, ghostly-looking skin. That is why so many women hide their sun-starved skins with face makeup. People who are deprived of the vital rays of the sun have a half-dead look. They are actually dying for want of solar energy! Weak, ailing, anemic people are usually sun-starved and, in our opinion, many people are sick simply because they are starving for sunshine.

The rays of the sun are powerful germicides! As the skin imbibes more of these rays, it stores up enormous amounts of this germ-killing energy. The gentle sun provides a remedy for the nervous person filled with anxiety, worry, stresses and strains. When these tense people lie in the early morning or late afternoon gentle sunshine, its healing rays give them what the nerves and body are crying out for . . . and that is gentle relaxation!

There is no substitute for Good Health!
Those who possess health are richer than kings! – Paul C. Bragg, ND, PhD.

What sculpture is to a block of marble, education is to the mind and soul.
– Joseph Addison, "The Spectator Newspaper", England, 1711

Chlorophyll is Miracle Liquid Sunshine

Gentle sunshine is a soothing tonic, a stimulant and above all, the Great Healer! As you bask in the warm, gentle sunshine (not the hot afternoon sun), millions of nerve endings absorb the energy from the sun and transform it so the body's nervous system can use it.

Perform this experiment to determine the value of sunshine in the matter of life and death. Find a beautiful lawn, where the grass is like a green carpet. Cover up a small space of that beautiful lawn with a piece of wood or a small box. Day by day you will soon notice that the beautiful grass that once was full of plant blood, precious chlorophyll, will fade and turn a sickly yellow. Tragically, it withers and dies – death by sun starvation! The same thing happens in your body without the sun's life-giving rays and without an abundance of sun-ripened foods such as organic fruits, vegetables and their fresh juices.

We must have the direct gentle rays of the sun on our bodies and at least 60% to 70% percent of the food we eat must have been ripened by the sun's rays. When we eat fresh, organically grown fruits and vegetables, we absorb the blood of the plant – chlorophyll. This life-giving chlorophyll is the solar energy that the plant has absorbed from the sun, the richest, most nourishing health food you can put in your body. Green plants and vegetables alone possess the secret of how to capture this powerful solar energy and pass it on to man and every other living creature. When you put sunshine on the outside of your body and eat ample sun-grown, organic fruits and vegetables, you are going to glow with more super health! But these powerful, natural remedies must be taken in small doses at the beginning, because your sun-starved body can't absorb too much at first.

God gave His creatures light and air and water open to the skies;
Man locks himself in a stifling lair and wonders why his brother dies.
– Oliver W. Holmes, Associate Justice to U.S. Supreme Court, 1902-1932

Freedom and progress rest in man's continual searching for truth.
Truth is the summit of being. – Ralph Waldo Emerson

Gentle Sunbathing Works Miracles!

When you begin sunbathing, start with short time periods until you condition your body to take more. The best time for beginners to start taking 10 and 15 minute sunbaths is in the early morning sunshine until 10 a.m. or late afternoon sunshine after 3 p.m. Between 11 and 3 we usually avoid stronger, burning rays. (*We wear straw hats.*)

The same caution should be taken when eating the sun-ripened raw fruits and vegetables. The average person who has been eating mainly cooked foods will find that if great amounts of raw fruits and vegetables suddenly enter into the body they can cause a reaction. It's wiser to gradually add more sun-ripened foods to the diet. Overdoses of solar energy, both outside and inside the body, are not wise. Regarding sun exposure, use good judgment and caution. For sun (skin) protection make a green herb (non-caffeine) tea, then bottle, apply to skin when needed.

Doctor Healing Sunshine Saved Bragg's Life!

When my father was diagnosed with tuberculosis at 16, three TB Sanitariums later, the best TB doctors in USA declared his case *hopeless and incurable!* Yet, by the grace of God, he was led to Dr. August Rollier of Leysin, Switzerland, the greatest living authority on heliotherapy (sun cure). High in the Swiss Alps, Dad's sick and wasted body was exposed to the gentle healing rays of the sun and was fed an abundance of natural, sun-ripened foods.

A healing miracle happened. In just two years he was transformed from a hopeless invalid to a vitally strong young man who radiated health! Throughout Paul Bragg's long, fulfilled life he was healthy, happy, powerful in sports and always enjoyed the great outdoors and the healing rays of the gentle sun on his body.

A wise man should consider that health is the greatest of human blessings! To learn how, by his own guidance, to learn from his illnesses and then change any unhealthy living habits to 100% healthy habits and start now!

Nature never deceives us; it's always we who deceive ourselves. – Rousseau

Laughter is a sunbeam for the soul. – Thomas Mann, author, "The Magic Mountain"

Enjoy God's own Sunshine for Super Health

That is why my father and I have always loved God's own precious sunshine. That's why we made our main home in California, the great sunshine state. We have an organic farm in Santa Barbara near the ocean where we get the benefits of the clean air and sunshine. We also live part-time in Hawaii so we can visit with the Bragg readers who visit our free Bragg Exercise Class (see page iii) at famous Waikiki Beach. The class is 6 days a week and it's fun to exercise in the fresh clean ocean air. We enjoy our students who come from all over the world. Seek fresh, clean air, gentle sunshine and organic sun-kissed foods, then soon super health will leap out and be yours to treasure throughout a long, ever youthful, productive, happy life!

Visit: *www.BraggHawaiiExercise.com*

Kind hearts are the gardens,
Kind thoughts are the roots,
Kind words are the flowers,
Kind deeds are the fruits.
Take care of your garden,
And keep out the weeds,
Fill it with sunshine,
Kind words and kind deeds."

– Henry Wadsworth Longfellow

May flowers always line your path and sunshine light your day.
May songbirds serenade your every step along the way.
May a rainbow run beside you in a sky that's always blue.
And may happiness fill your heart each day your whole life through.

– Old Irish Blessing

Those who bring sunshine to the lives of others
cannot keep it from themselves. – James Matthew Barrie

Wherever you go, no matter what the weather,
always bring your own sunshine. – Anthony J. D'Angelo

Chapter 24

Keep Oxygen – The Invisible Staff of Life Flowing for Life

Breathing is one of the most essential activities of life. We have already considered how, unlike with drinking or eating, we can live for only a very few short minutes without breathing! The work of bringing oxygen into the lungs and getting it into the bloodstream where it will be sent to nourish every cell of the body is the very basis of human life! It is for this reason that my father developed The Bragg Super Power Breathing. It is more than just a technique for better breathing, what we are describing to you in this book is a whole philosophy of breathing. By your mastering The Bragg Super Power Breathing you will maximize your lungs' capacity for oxygenating your body and your capacity for making use of this vital nourishment, the invisible staff of life!

But even The Bragg Super Power Breathing can't guarantee that you will always be getting the oxygen you need. Emergency rescue personnel, medics, lifeguards and others around the country and around the world can attest to this: even the healthiest, fittest, most vital of people can suddenly and unexpectedly be threatened with oxygen starvation. Unlike the slow suffocation most people suffer because of bad breathing habits, sudden suffocation refers to dangers of choking, drowning, asthma attacks and other events that can deprive a person of needed, life-giving oxygen. (See pages 200-203)

The Bragg Healthy Lifestyle, along with Super Power Breathing (SPB), can go a long way in helping asthmatics overcome dangerous effects of their breathing condition, though the onset of an asthmatic attack still threatens the SPB breather with oxygen deprivation. Likewise, the choking or drowning victim who is a SPB will suffocate just the same, unless the object or water is removed.

Breathe deeply and allow yourself to be filled with life energizing oxygen for a vital life filled with health, energy, laughter, peace and love.
– Patricia Bragg, ND, PhD., Pioneer Health Crusader

The Heimlich Maneuver Jumpstarts the Lungs

My father and I want to do all we can to ensure that all people are able to get all the oxygen they need. We have even included how to get the asthma or choking and drowning accident victims breathing again, page 203.

Many of you are familiar with the famous Heimlich Maneuver* as a technique for saving choking victims. Since 1974, this procedure has saved more than 70,000 lives just in the United States. This maneuver, developed by Dr. Henry J. Heimlich, is performed by pressing upward on the diaphragm. This compresses the lungs, causing a flow of air that helps push the choking object out that is blocking the airway. Recent evidence and research has suggested the Heimlich Maneuver is effective in restoring breathing in more emergency situations than just choking. Our friends, Dr. Heimlich along with his wife Jane Murray Heimlich (*daughter of famous Arthur and Katherine Murray who taught America to dance)*, have dedicated their lives to educating the world about the life-saving Heimlich Maneuver. See: *HeimlichHeroes.org*

Heimlich Helps Save Drowning Victims

In more than 90% of drowning cases, the victim's lungs fill with fluid. In this situation, it is imperative that the fluid be expelled quickly – because after four or five minutes the likelihood of brain damage increases. Just getting someone out of the water has not changed their condition – if they still have fluid in their lungs their condition is the same as if they were still under water. In all the studies on drowning since 1933, none showed that mouth-to-mouth resuscitation saved drowning victims without first draining water from their lungs! This is common sense, air cannot get into water-filled lungs!

The Heimlich Maneuver expels water from the lungs of drowning victims in six to nine seconds – with two to four Heimlich applications! And unlike CPR, when applied correctly, Heimlich is safe and easily mastered by person new to procedure. NOTE: Gently hold babies upside down to drain water out, then do Heimlich Maneuver.

* Visit webs: www.HeimlichInstitute.org or www.HeimlichHeroes.org

CPR unfortunately often causes rib fractures, lung punctures, internal bleeding and injuries of all sorts. In one study of 323 people who died after receiving CPR, 17% of the people likely died of injuries caused by CPR! Adding to danger of using too strong CPR in asphyxiation situations, another study finds in 86% of cases, a drowning (or choking) victim vomits after resuscitation by CPR. Vomiting can cause airway blockage and death if not cleared. (It happened to a friend. Most ambulances carry airway tubes for this, sadly his didn't.) In contrast, less than 3% of cases vomited after the safer Heimlich Maneuver.

Heimlich Maneuver Stops Asthma Attacks

More cases are being documented of the effectiveness of the Heimlich Maneuver in stopping asthma attacks. As Dr. Heimlich explains, *"We started receiving reports from people who had suffered severe, almost deadly asthma attacks. The people who were with them didn't have any idea what to do. Off the top of their heads, they used the Heimlich Maneuver. They just tried it to help,"* he says, *"and immediately, a miracle happened, the asthma attack stopped!"*

When the diaphragm of an asthma attack victim is pushed up with the Heimlich Maneuver (whether self-applied or not), the lungs become compressed. When this happens, trapped air is forcibly expelled and air flow carries away the mucus plugs that started the attack. After the Maneuver, airway is cleared and prayerfully asthma attack ends!

When the Heimlich is performed on asthmatics, do it gently, because you are expelling mucus and trapped air – not a stuck food object or lungs full of water. There's good evidence this maneuver can also prevent an asthma attack from occurring. Studies show applying procedure on regular basis helps keep lungs free of mucus that can plug up airway and bring on asthma attack. It's best to avoid mucus forming dairy and unhealthy food products!

Anyone Can Be a Heimlich Hero – *From professional baseball stars to grade-school students, anyone can step in and save someone from choking to death. You don't have to be an adult or a doctor. You won't need muscles and strength. With the right knowledge and know-how, you can prevent a choking death.* Visit web: www.HeimlichHeroes.org

Heimlich Maneuver – It is Life-Saving!

Dr. Henry J. Heimlich with Patricia Bragg in Honolulu

In 1974, Dr. Heimlich published findings on what was to become the Heimlich Maneuver®. A week later, the first choking victim was saved by the method. Since its introduction, Heimlich Maneuver has saved over 70,000 people in the United States alone from choking or drowning.

"I have saved two lives doing the Heimlich myself – one man in Sydney restaurant choking on meat, another young man at Disneyland Restaurant in Orlando, Florida." – Dr. Patricia

Take the advice of the National Pool and Water Park Association, learn the Heimlich Maneuver* – it's the resuscitation technique they now recommend as first step in treating drowning victims. Results prove it works!

*Heimlich Institute, 311 Straight Street, Cincinnati, OH 45219 (513) 559-2100 or visit on web at: www.HeimlichInstitute.org

Even Young People Can Learn to do the Heimlich

The ***Heimlich Heroes Program*** (*HeimlichHeroes.org*) was developed to teach 6th grade students the life-saving Heimlich Maneuver. The Program is specifically designed to instruct young people how to do the Heimlich Maneuver. The Program teaches them how to: recognize signs of choking; understand how to respond if a person is actually choking; and learn ways to help prevent or minimize risks of choking.

The *Heimlich Heroes Program* **is instructional, valuable, interactive and fun.** That's what the program is all about. It teaches a life-saving technique; empowers young people to see themselves as potential heroes; links learning experiences with real-world events; features hands-on material and online training; enables young people to react confidently during an emergency situation; keeps the students engaged and energized; increases student confidence, independence and self-esteem; it is easy to use and free to the user.
Heimlich Heroes believes anyone can save a life.

202

Heimlich Life-Saving Maneuver

First Aid for Choking and Drowning Victims and Sufferers of Asthma Breathing Attacks
(With Victim Standing or Sitting)

Standing in pool or water, buoyancy of water helps lighten the victim's weight.

Save Drowning victim the
HEIMLICH MANEUVER
You can't get air into lungs
until you get water out!

I saved 2 choking victims – strangers at restaurants 1 in Florida, 1 in Sydney Australia, with Heimlich.
– Dr. Patricia

Hold Baby Down

1. Stand behind the victim and wrap your arms firmly around their upper waist.

2. Place the thumb side of your fist strongly against the victim's abdomen, slightly above the navel and below the rib cage.

3. Grasp your fist with other hand and press your fist into the abdomen with a quick upward thrust. Repeat until food/water is expelled. Do this more gently for asthma attacks.

4. If the victim is sitting, stand behind their chair and perform Maneuver in the same manner.

5. After victim has been revived and saved, have them see doctor.

Note: If you start to choke when alone and help is not available, then you should self-administer this Maneuver yourself. Many have had too, and it works!

First Aid when Victim has Collapsed and Can't be Lifted, Follow This Procedure:

1. Lay victim on back. Face them, kneel astride hips and thighs. (with babies, hold upside down to let water out, then do Heimlich.)

2. With one hand on top of another, place heel of bottom hand on abdomen above the navel and just below the rib-cage.

3. Press into the victim's abdomen with a quick upward thrust. Repeat as often as necessary.

4. Should victim vomit, (some do), quickly tilt head to side and wipe out vomit from mouth to prevent blocking of throat airway. (Use airway tube if necessary – keep one in first aid kit.)

5. After food, water, etc. is out, it's best a doctor check the victim.

Shortness of Breath in Heart Attack Victims

Shortness of breath is common symptom for people with heart failure. Shortness of breath occurs because blood in the body backs up in the blood vessels that return blood from the lungs to the heart due to the heart not pumping blood out of the heart effectively! This causes fluid to leak into lungs. If you experience SEVERE and persistent shortness of breath you should call for emergency treatment immediately.

Most people who experience cardiac arrest at home, work or in public die because they don't receive immediate CPR from someone on the scene! As a bystander, don't be afraid. Your actions can only help! The chances of surviving cardiac arrest with good brain function are better when bystanders focus on Hands Only CPR. The hands-only technique may be more effective than conventional CPR in the early phase of sudden cardiac arrest, which may be all that is needed if an automated external defibrillator (AED) is available nearby.✶

Hands-Only™ CPR Can and is Saving Lives!

If you witness a person collapse having a heart attack – American Heart Association recommends you call 911 – FAST, then start to continuously push hard and fast in middle of chest, ideal 100 pushes a minute with force to make chest go down & up 1^1/$_2$ inches. See video: *HandsOnlyCPR.org.* If the heart can be kept going, medications usually help strengthen the heart enough so slowly the body can re-route blood to damaged heart muscle through other tiny vessels! This re-routing miracle process, called collateral circulation, helps keep many heart-attack victims alive and recovering!

Million Hearts® is a national initiative to prevent 1 million heart attacks *and strokes by 2017. Million Hearts® brings together communities, health systems, nonprofit organizations, federal agencies, and private-sector from across the country to fight heart disease and stroke and to improve care and empower Americans to make heart-healthy choices!* – See web: MillionHearts.hhs.gov.

✶**Automated External Defibrillator (AED) Offers Fast Miracle . . .** *for victims of sudden cardiac arrest! Studies say that survival rate for those who received their first defibrillation shock, no more than 3 minutes after collapse has 74%, as opposed to 49%, survival rate. The FAA has decided most passenger planes will carry an AED. Medical Centers, big businesses, universities, schools, cruise ships, etc. will soon have one in their first aid kits too.* – nejm.org

Heart Smart Devices and Supplies, visit web: HeartSmart.com

Chapter 25

Healthy Alternatives to Help with Breathing Problems

- Nutritional, Herbal & Water Therapy
- Massage • Acupuncture • Chiropractic
- Natural Alternative Therapies

Don't Accept Breathing Problems – Solve Them

The healthiest, best thing to do instead of taking drugs for asthma, sinus, bronchitis, COPD and other breathing problems is to seek natural remedies to correct any problems! Drugs should never be the main method of seeking a cure. These drugs and applications are commonly called "maintenance drugs". Even this is misleading because the problems they supposedly relieve often get worse over time. Sadly. not to mention the many other side effects they have on the entire body!

The three prominent types of drugs for sinus/asthma problems in the medical field are: bronchodilators, (see pages 85-88) anti-inflammatories and antihistamines. Although the first two can supply some relief during attacks by opening narrowed breathing pathways, they are very dangerous and ill-advised. A study of bronchodilators, (drug puffers) in New Zealand found that their habit forming use brought an increased risk of asthma-related deaths and injury. Antihistamines, on the other hand, really promise no relief to asthma sufferers, even in the short-term. Their effect is merely to dry up mucus secretions and replace the aggravating plugs of thick mucus with dried, clogging crusts of mucus.

For a healthy nose, it's essential to live The Bragg Healthy Lifestyle. Practice this lifestyle formula for good physical and mental health! A healthy head and body are necessary preconditions to a healthy, happy nose! (see pages 35-41)

According to recent medical studies more people suffer from a condition called multiple chemical sensitivity. Now it is more crucial that you and your family practice natural healthy living habits to stay healthy!

Pollution and Wrong Diet Affects Breathing

In addition, if you live in a polluted area, or if your sinuses are already damaged from the hard work of protecting your lungs, buy a high-efficiency, charcoal particulate HEPA air filtration system. This pre-filters the air your sinuses will filter, making your nose's job easier. Also have one for your home, office and car (see page 119).

You must also be intelligent about your allergies. If you know you are allergic to particular substances, take precautions to avoid them. If you suspect allergies, take the necessary steps to learn what's affecting you. The most common allergens are mold spores, animal hair and dander, toxic house dust, mites, pollens and even carpet and paint chemicals, etc. Food allergies are also a frequent source of allergic respiratory reactions (see page 39-40).

With long-term relief in mind, stay informed about the effective alternative therapies available today. The most sensible therapy to practice, no matter what the health complaint, is *Nutritional Therapy*. When it comes to sinus problems it's most important to avoid dairy products of all kinds. Dairy foods are unhealthy for the nose and the whole body. Dairy proteins often mimic allergens by causing the nose and throat airway passages to swell. They also increase mucus production. This in turn causes sinus discomfort and can give rise to dangerous bacterial conditions. If you are a snorer (see page 99-101) or a sufferer of any sinus condition you will especially benefit from a no-dairy diet. Try it – prove it to yourself!

In addition to healthy living and avoiding all dairy, you can relieve sinusitis symptoms and bolster the health of your nose by using *Herbal Therapy* such as: licorice, anise and horehound, Brigham tea, mint, echinacea, fenugreek, goldenseal, lobelia, marshmallow, mullein, red clover and rose hips (see page 38). Herbs are available in teas, capsules or tablets. Medicinal herbs, soaked in a cloth poultice (hot), can provide relief for sore, congested areas. (Example: old fashion mustard chest pack for chest colds.)

The Lord gives strength to those who are weary. – Isaiah 40:29

Perfect health is above gold; a sound body before riches. – Solomon

No matter what therapies you practice, consider *Water Therapy*, a health essential! Never fail to drink at least 8 tall glasses of purified/distilled water daily. This helps your mucus membranes and sinuses efficiently filter and dispose of any contaminants that you breathe in the air. In this book we have continued to inform you of all the various health alternatives for your health!

Also try this soothing detox shower: apply Bragg Olive Oil to skin, alternate hot and cold water, every 2-3 minutes. Massage body while under hot, filtered spray. Garden hose massage is great in summer or anytime. Hot detox soak bath (diabetics use warm water) 20 minutes with cup of Epsom salts or apple cider vinegar. This soak helps pull out toxins by creating an artificial fever cleanse. Web: *HolisticOnLine.com/Hydrotherapy.htm*

Healthy Alternative Massage Techniques

REIKI A Japanese form of massage that means "Universal Life Energy." Reiki Massage helps the body to detoxify, then re-balance and heal itself. Discovered in the ancient Sutra manuscripts by Dr. Mikao Usui in 1922. Web: *Reiki.org*

ROLFING Developed by Ida Rolf in the 1930's in the U.S. Rolfing is also called structural processing and postural release, or structural dynamics. It is based on the concept that distortions (accidents, injuries, falls, etc.) and the effects of gravity on the body cause upsets and long-term stress in the body. Rolfing helps to achieve balance and improved body posture. Methods involve the use of stretching, deep tissue massage, and relaxation techniques to loosen old injuries and break bad movement and posture patterns. Web: *Rolf.org*

TRAGERING Founded by Dr. Milton Trager M.D., who was inspired at age 18 by Paul C. Bragg to become a doctor. It is a mind-body learning method that involves gentle shaking and rocking, allowing the body to let go, releasing tensions and lengthening the muscles for more body peace and health. Tragering can do miraculous healing where needed in the body frame, muscles and the entire body. Web: *www.Trager.com*

MASSAGE & AROMATHERAPY works two ways: the essence (aroma) relaxes, as does healing massages. Essential oils are extracted from flowers, leaves, roots, seeds and barks. These are usually massaged into the skin, inhaled or used in a bath for their ability to relax, soothe and heal. The oils, used for centuries to treat numerous ailments, are revitalizing and energizing for the body and mind. Example: Tiger balm, MSM, echinacea and arnica help relieve muscle aches. (Avoid skin creams and lotions with mineral oil – it clogs the skin's pores.) Use these natural oils for the skin: almond, avocado, and I use Bragg Organic Olive Oil (page 240) and mix with aromatic essential oils: rosemary, lavender, rose, jasmine, sandalwood or lemon-balm, etc. – 6 oz. oil and 4 drops of an essential oil. Web: *NAHA.org*

SELF MASSAGE Paul C. Bragg often said, "You can be your own best massage therapist, even if you have only one good hand." Near-miraculous health improvements have been achieved by victims of accidents or strokes in bringing life back to afflicted parts of their own bodies by self-massage and even vibrators. Treatments can be day or night, almost continual. Self-massage also helps achieve relaxation at day's end. Families and friends can learn and exchange massages; it's a wonderful sharing experience. Remember, babies love and thrive with daily massages, start from birth. Family pets also love soothing, healing touch of massages. Web: *RD.com/health/wellness/learn-the-art-of-self-massage/*

SHIATSU MASSAGE Japanese form of massage that applies pressure from fingers, hands, elbows and even knees along the same points as acupuncture. This technique can bring relief for the asthmatic. Although it bears some similarity to needle acupuncture, Shaitsu uses finger-pressure, like Acupressure Therapy to stimulate the body's own rehabilitative functions. Shiatsu Therapy has become popular for the victims of sinus and allergy discomfort. Shiatsu has been used in Asia for centuries to relieve pain, common ills, muscle stress and to aid lymphatic circulation. Web: *Shiatsu.org*

Where there is great love there are always miracles.
– Willa Cather, Pulitzer Prize-winning author

SPORTS MASSAGE An important health support system for professional and amateur athletes. Sports massage improves circulation and mobility to injured tissue, enables athletes to recover more rapidly from myofascial injury, reduces muscle soreness and chronic strain patterns. Soft tissues are freed of trigger points and adhesions, thus contributing to improvement of peak neuromuscular functioning and athletic performance.

SWEDISH MASSAGE One of the oldest and most widely used massage techniques. This deep body massage soothes and promotes healthy circulation and is a great way to loosen and relax tight muscles before and after exercise. See web: *MassageDen.com/Swedish-Massage.shtml*

Alternative Health Therapies for Healing Try Them – They Work Miracles!

Explore these wonderful natural methods of healing your body. Finally over 600 Medical Schools in U.S. are teaching Healthy Alternative Therapies. Please check the websites. Seek and choose the best healing techniques for you:

ACUPUNCTURE/ACUPRESSURE **Acupuncture** directs and rechannels body energy by inserting hair-thin needles (*use only disposable*) at specific points on the body. This professional placement of needles often can provide relief from airway spasms and encourage passages to dilate, permitting greater flow of air. It helps to relieve the complaints of asthma and sinus problems. It's also used for pain, backaches, migraines and general health and body dysfunctions. Used in Asia for centuries, acupuncture is safe, virtually painless and has no side effects. **Acupressure** is based on the same principles and uses finger pressure and massage rather than needles. Websites offer info, check them out: *AcupunctureToday.com* or *Acupressure.com*

Caring hands have healing life-force energy . . . babies love and thrive with daily massages and cuddles. Family pets love soothing, healing touches. Everyone benefits from healing massages and treatments!
– Patricia Bragg, ND, PhD., Pioneer Health & Lifestyle Educator

---

Perhaps the most valuable result of all education is the ability to make yourself do the thing you have to do, when it ought to be done, as it ought to be done, whether you like it or not!

209

CHIROPRACTIC was founded in Davenport, Iowa in 1885 by Daniel David Palmer. There are now many schools in the U.S., and graduates are joining Health Practitioners in all nations of the world to share healing techniques. Chiropractic is popular and the largest U.S. healing profession benefitting literally millions! Chiropractic Therapy has shown to provide relief by stimulating the nerves that control the lungs. The nerves that send messages to the lungs are located on the spine just below the neck and can be manipulated for increased stimulation. These procedures can also have beneficial effects on the diaphragm. Some practitioners can even make adjustments on some of the small bones and cartilage of the nose for increased breathing comfort. Treatment also involves soft tissue, spinal and body adjustment to free the nervous system of interferences with normal body function. Its concern is the functional integrity of the musculoskeletal system. In addition to manual methods, chiropractors use physical therapy modalities exercise, health and nutritional guidance. Web: *ChiroWeb.com*

F. MATTHIAS ALEXANDER TECHNIQUE These lessons help end improper use of neuromuscular system and bring body posture back into balance. Eliminates psycho-physical interferences, helps release long-held tension, and aids in re-establishing muscle tone. The Alexander Technique helps people unlearn bad physical habits and return to a balanced state of rest and poise in which the body is well-aligned. Web: *AlexanderTechnique.com*

FELDENKRAIS METHOD Dr. Moshé Feldenkrais founded this method in the late 1940s. This Method leads to improved posture and helps create ease and efficiency of body movement. The practitioner directs attention to habitual movement patterns which are inefficient or strained, and teaches new patterns using gentle, slow, repeated movements. Web: *www.Feldenkrais.com*

Author's Comment: We have personally sampled many of these Alternative Therapies. It's estimated America's health care costs are over $2.9 trillion. It's more important now to be responsible for our own health! This includes seeking dedicated holistic health practitioners to keep us well by inspiring us to practice prevention! These Alternative Healing Therapies are also popular and getting results: aromatherapy, Ayurvedic, biofeedback, color, guided imagery, herbs, hyperbaric oxygen, music, meditation, magnets, saunas, tai chi, Qi gong, Pilates, Rebounder, Bemer, yoga, etc. Explore and be open to improving your earthly temple for a healthy, happier, longer life. *Seek & find the best for your body, mind & soul.* – Patricia Bragg, ND, PhD.

Healing Natural Therapy & Healthy Lifestyle

HOMEOPATHY In the 1800's, Dr. Samuel Hahnemann developed homeopathy. Patients are treated with "micro" doses of remedies found in nature to trigger the body's own defenses. This homeopathic principle is a safe and nontoxic remedy and is the #1 alternative therapy in Europe and Britain because it is inexpensive, seldom has any side effects, and usually brings fast results. Web: *Homeopathic.org*

NATUROPATHY Brought to America by Dr. Benedict Lust this treatment uses diet, herbs, homeopathy, fasting, exercise, hydrotherapy, manipulation and sunlight. (Dr. Paul Bragg graduated from Dr. Lust's first School of Naturopathy in U.S. Now there are 8 schools.) Practitioners work with your body to restore health naturally. They reject surgery and drugs except as a last resort. Web: *Naturopathic.org*

OSTEOPATHY The first School of Osteopathy was founded in 1892 by Dr. Andrew Taylor Still. There are now 31 U.S. colleges. Treatment involves soft tissue, spinal and body adjustments that free the nervous system from interferences that can cause illness. Healing by adjustment also includes good nutrition, physical therapies, proper breathing and good posture. Dr. Still's premise: if the body structure is altered or abnormal, then proper body function is altered and can cause pain and illness. Web: *www.Osteopathic.org*

REFLEXOLOGY OR ZONE THERAPY Founded by Eunice Ingham, author of *Stories The Feet Can Tell* (book available *amazon.com*), inspired by a Bragg Health Crusade when she was 17. Reflexology helps the body and organs by removing crystalline deposits from reflex areas (nerve endings) of feet and hands through deep pressure massage. Primitive reflexology originated in China and Egypt and Native American Indians and Kenyans self-practiced it for centuries. Reflexology activates the body's flow of healing and energy by dislodging deposits. Visit Eunice Ingham and nephew Dwight Byer's website: *Reflexology-usa.net*

SKIN BRUSHING daily is wonderful for circulation, toning, cleansing and healing. Use a dry vegetable brush (never nylon) and brush lightly. Helps purify lymph so it's able to detoxify your blood and tissues. Removes old skin cells, uric acid crystals and toxic wastes that come up through skin's pores. Use loofah sponge for variety in shower or tub.

Health is Your Birthright – Protect and Treasure It!

This is a priceless health book. Please read and re-read this book until you absorb every health nugget it contains. Remember that you and you alone control your life, your health and the way you look, act, think and feel! Health comes from the inside out. You can be patched up after being stricken with disease, sickness and physical pain, but 100% true, robust, vital health comes from good *health habits!* This book shows you how to turn away from damaging, unhealthy lifestyle habits that careless, wrong living promotes in this hectic, fast-food age!

It is up to you to apply the intelligence that our Creator gave you. We teach simple, healthy living. You now have a treasure of knowledge of how to create a healthier, more joyful life through living this simple, healthy lifestyle. Have faith in yourself, start now!

Your health depends on how healthy your lifestyle is, the way you conduct yourself each hour, each day, each week, each month and each year! You are the sum total of your habits! It is true that your body can take a lot of punishment from your bad habits. Sure, you can smoke, drink, eat dead, devitalized foods and apparently look and feel fine. Yes, for a while . . . but sooner or later you will have to balance your debts with Mother Nature! And when something breaks and you have heart trouble or one of hundreds of other life and health destroying miseries, it may be too late! It may mean years of painful living – or sadly it may mean a quick death.

We have no supernatural power to prevent or cure disease. That power is in your body! Your body is self-cleansing and self-healing when given a chance. We can only come to you as health teachers, to tell you in a simple way what living this healthy lifestyle will do for you. You have the knowledge; it's now up to you to apply the intelligence that our Creator gave you! **Living The Bragg Healthy Lifestyle is simply good common sense.**

Knowing these teachings will mean true life and good health for you.
– Proverbs 4:22

With your new awareness, understanding and sincere commitment of how to live The Bragg Healthy Lifestyle – you can now live a longer, healthier life to 120 years! *(Gen. 6:3)*

God bless you and your family and may He give you the strength, the courage and the patience to win your battle to re-enter the Healthy Garden of Eden while you are still living here on Earth with more years to enjoy it all!

With Blessings of Health, Peace, Joy and Love,

Health Crusaders Paul C. Bragg and daughter Patricia traveled the world spreading health, inspiring millions to renew and revitalize their health.
– 3 John 2
– Genesis 6:3

The Bragg books are written to inspire and guide you to health, fitness and longevity. Remember, the book you don't read won't help. So please reread Bragg Books and live The Bragg Healthy Lifestyle to enjoy a healthy fulfilled life!

I never suspected that I would have to learn how to live – that there were specific disciplines and ways of seeing the world that I had to master before I could awaken to a simple, healthy, happy, uncomplicated life.
– Dan Millman, Author of "The Way of the Peaceful Warrior" • www.danmillman.com
A Bragg fan and admirer since his Stanford University coaching days.

A truly good book teaches me better than to just read it,
I must soon lay it down and commence living in its wisdom.
What I began by reading, I must finish by acting! – Henry David Thoreau

GO ORGANIC! DON'T PANIC!   GUARD YOUR TOTAL HEALTH

FROM THE AUTHORS

This book was written for You! It can be your passport to a healthy, long, vital life. We in the Alternative Health Therapies join hands in one common objective – promoting a high standard of health for everyone. Healthy Nutrition points the way – which is Mother Nature and God's Way. This book teaches you how to work with them, not against them! Health Doctors, Therapists Nurses, Teachers and Caregivers are becoming more dedicated than ever before to keeping their patients healthy and fit. This book was written to emphasize the great needed importance of healthy lifestyle living for health and longevity, close to Mother Nature and God.

Statements in this book are scientific health findings, known facts of physiology and biological therapeutics. Paul C. Bragg practiced natural methods of living for over 80 years with highly beneficial results, knowing that they were safe and of great value. His daughter Patricia lectured and co-authored Bragg Health Books with him and continues carrying on Bragg Health Crusades and Bragg Foundation.

Paul C. Bragg and daughter Patricia express their opinions solely as Public Health Educators and Health Crusaders. They offer no cure for disease. Only the body has the ability to cure a person. Experts may disagree with some of the statements made in this book. However, such statements are considered to be factual, based on the long-time experience of dedicated pioneer Health Crusaders Paul C. Bragg and Patricia Bragg. If you suspect you have a medical problem, please always seek qualified health care professionals to help you make the healthiest, wisest and best-informed choices!

Count your blessings daily *while you do your 30 to 45 minute brisk walks and exercises with these affirmations – health! strength! youth! vitality! peace! laughter! humility! understanding! forgiveness! joy! and love for eternity! and soon all these qualities will come flooding and bouncing into your life! With blessings of super health, peace and love to you, our dear friends, our readers. – Patricia Bragg, ND, PhD., Health Crusader*

Oxygen is the main nutrient of the body. When we improve our oxygen intake, we enhance our immune system and the body's ability to detoxify and stay healthy for a long life. – Dr. Michael Schachter, Columbia University

If I were to name the three most precious resources of life, I would say books, friends and nature; and the greatest of these, at least the most constant and always at hand is Mother Nature and God. – John Burroughs

214

KEEP HEALTHY & YOUTHFUL BIOLOGICALLY WITH EXERCISE & GOOD NUTRITION

Always remember you have the following important reasons for following The Bragg Healthy Lifestyle:

- The ironclad laws of Mother Nature and God.
- Your common sense, which tells you that you are doing right.
- Your aim to make your health better and your life longer.
- Your resolve to prevent illness so that you may enjoy life.
- Make an art of healthy living; you will be youthful at any age.
- You will retain your faculties and be hale, hearty, active and useful far beyond the ordinary length of years.
- You will also possess superior mental and physical powers!

WANTED – For Robbing Health & Life

KILLER Saturated Fats	CHOKER Hydrogenated Fats
CLOGGER Salt	DEADEYED Devitalized Foods
DOPEY Caffeine	HARD WATER Inorganic Minerals
PLUGGER Frying Pan	JERKY Turbulent Emotions
DEATH-DEALER Drugs	CRAZY Alcohol
GREASY Overweight	SMOKEY Tobacco
HOGGY Overeating	LOAFER Laziness

What Wise Men Say

Wisdom does not show itself so much in precept as in life – a firmness of mind and mastery of the appetite. – Seneca

Govern well thy appetite, lest Sin surprise thee, and her black attendant, Death. – Milton

Our prayers should be for a sound mind in a healthy body. – Juvenal

I saw few die of hunger – of eating, a hundred thousand.
– Ben Franklin

Your health is your wealth.
– Paul C. Bragg, ND, PhD.

Health is a blessing that money cannot buy. – Izaak Walton

The natural healing force within us is the greatest force in getting well.
– Hippocrates, Father of Medicine, 400 BC

Of all the knowledge, the one most worth having is knowledge about health! The first requisite of a good life is to be a healthy person. – Herbert Spencer

215

THE MIRACLES OF APPLE CIDER VINEGAR FOR A STRONGER, LONGER, HEALTHIER LIFE

> **The old adage is true:**
> *"An apple a day
> keeps the doctor away."*

- Helps promote a youthful skin and vibrant healthy body
- Helps remove artery plaque, infections and body toxins
- Helps fight germs, viruses, bacteria and mold naturally
- Helps retard old age onset in humans, pets and farm animals
- Helps regulate calcium metabolism
- Helps keep blood the right consistency
- Helps regulate women's menstruation, relieves PMS, and UTI
- Helps normalize urine pH, relieving frequent urge to urinate
- Helps digestion, assimilation and helps balance the pH
- Helps protect against food poisoning and even brings relief if you do get it
- Helps relieve sore throats, laryngitis and throat tickles and cleans out throat and gum toxins
- Helps detox the body so sinus, asthma and flu sufferers can breathe easier and more normally
- Helps banish acne, athlete's foot, soothes burns, sunburns
- Helps prevent itching scalp, baldness, and dry hair
- Helps banish dandruff, rashes, and shingles
- Helps fight arthritis and helps remove crystals and toxins from joints, tissues, organs and entire body
- Helps control and normalize body weight

– Paul C. Bragg, ND, PhD., Health Crusader,
Originator of Health Stores

Our sincere blessings to you, dear friends, who make our lives so worthwhile and fulfilled by reading our teachings on natural living as our Creator laid down for us to follow. He wants us to follow the simple path of natural living. This is what we teach in our books and health crusades worldwide. Our prayers reach out to you and your loved ones for the best in health and happiness. We must follow these wise laws He has laid down for us, so we can reap this precious health physically, mentally, emotionally and spiritually!

***HAVE AN APPLE
HEALTHY LIFE!***

With Love,

Braggs Organic Raw Unfiltered Apple Cider Vinegar with the "Mother Enzyme" is #1 food I recommend to stop heartburn, gerds, gas, indigestion and for maintaining body's vital acid-alkaline balance and digestion.
– Gabriel Cousens, M.D., Author, "Conscious Eating"

Praises and Testimonials for The Bragg Healthy Lifestyle

If I could only have one condiment in my kitchen for the rest of my life, it would be Bragg's Liquid Aminos. I have been using it religiously for the past 12 years. Bragg Organic Apple Cider Vinegar is an important part of my daily health regimen, as well. Yum, Yum! – Amy Ragen, Granddaughter of McDonalds Founders', Ray & Joan Kroc

---

In 1998 I severely broke my left leg and doctors mended it with plates, screws and bolts. I developed staph and pus infections and sores on the bottom of my left foot. I had constant pain in my foot, ankle and knee. Since then I have had problems walking up and down stairs and kneeling was impossible. Then I started taking Bragg's Apple Cider Vinegar (2 Tbsps 3x a day). Two days after I started, the soreness in my knee disappeared and climbing the stairs is now pain free and all the other problems are gone!!! I never expected all these results, I give full credit to Bragg's Apple Cider Vinegar. Thank you. – Duke Jones, Ohio, Retired Police Officer

---

Love your Bragg All Natural Ginger & Sesame Salad Dressing, I bought here in Louisiana. It's delicious! Now I'm trying all your health products! I regained my health by eating organic foods and vegetables and taking supplements. I'm eating foods the way God created them and my body is thriving. Thanks for The Bragg Healthy Lifestyle – it's great!
– Candace Hawthorne, Metairie, Louisiana

Our great-grandmother will turn 100 in two weeks. She still kayaks, gardens, and even shovels her own snow covered driveway. For over 80 years, she had one recipe for life: 2 Tbsps Bragg ACV and 1 tsp of honey mixed into water. This is the secret, she says, to a life worth living. Five generations of our family will celebrate her 100th birthday with Bragg's Vinegar Drinks! Thank You!
– The Alvina Sharp Family, Minnesota

God promises miracle healings to people who fast and pray. – See Isaiah 58:6-9

217

Praises and Testimonials for The Bragg Healthy Lifestyle

Dr. Patricia Bragg is a dedicated Health Crusader and she shared her Bragg Healthy Lifestyle with millions of our TV and radio listeners. I take Bragg Vinegar faithfully every day for last 5 years. Thank you Patricia.
– Host George Noory • *www.CoastToCoastam.com*

Patricia, it was such an honor to meet you well over 15 years ago, before I was aware of the fabulous Bragg Health Crusades. Now I have been truly blessed by a more in-depth conversation with you about your life as the daughter of Paul C. Bragg and Bragg's amazing history. Thank you for all your knowledge of health and sharing it with the world. We are healthier and happier because of you!!
– With warm regards, Missy Woodward • *www.pcrm.org*
Physician Committee for Responsible Medicine, Wash. DC

I just wanted you to know that your Bragg ACV saved my cat's life. He was diagnosed with Cystitis (blockage of the urethra) which is common in cats. I spent $2500 in vet bills and 2 days after he came home, he stopped peeing and blocked up again. I read online to try Bragg ACV. I gave him ¼ tsp mixed with water, using syringe to feed it down his throat as he was not eating. Within the hour he peed 3 times in his litter box. He is healthier than ever and is even losing weight! He was 27 lbs. before he got sick, now healthy 19 lbs. Thanks to Bragg! – Ashley, Fort McMurray, Alberta, Canada

---

I'm a Champion Weight Lifter at Muscle Beach for 55 years and we are big Bragg fans. – Chris Baioa, Santa Monica, CA

I would like to thank you for teaching me how to take control of my health! I lost 55 pounds and I feel great! Bragg Health Books have showed me vitality, happiness and being close to Mother Nature. You both are real Health Crusaders for the World. Thanks. – Leonard Amato

---

I love Bragg Liquid Aminos on my food – it's great! – Thanks.
– Winning Coach Phil Jackson, for 11 years,
L.A. Lakers Championship Basketball Team

Praises and Testimonials for The Bragg Healthy Lifestyle

I have beat cancer twice. I lost my right kidney to cancer in 2002 and my left kidney in 2007. Part of my success was using Bragg's Health Products. Bragg Organic Apple Cider Vinegar with honey is the most effective and helps me so much. My brother Harvey Diamond was inspired by Bragg and wrote the book "Fit for Life". Thank you Paul and Patricia for your amazing Health Books and Products. – Mike Diamond

My "Fat Flush Plan" uses Bragg's Apple Cider Vinegar as a prime ingredient for seasoning and even cooking foods. We find that blood sugar becomes normalized and individuals can digest protein so much more effectively with Apple Cider Vinegar. It also provides the correct acid to compensate for the epidemic low stomach acid which is contributing to obesity, lack of proper calcium and iron absorption and protein malabsorption. Of course, I only recommend the best – Bragg Organic Apple Cider Vinegar.
– Ann Louise Gittleman, Ph.D., C.N.S. • *annlouise.com*
Author of 30 books on Health and Healing

Translating your "Apple Cider Vinegar" Book into Spanish has changed my outlook on life! I can never thank Patricia and her father enough! I was recently diagnosed with pre-diabetes and my fibromyalgia was flaring up. I was overweight and on high blood pressure medication. I started using Bragg's ACV and my blood pressure stabilized without pills! I got so excited I tried the other precepts in the book – eliminating coffee, sugar and white flour. I cut back on my meat consumption and ate organic raw veggies and fruits. Soon, I felt 15 years younger. I lost 10 pounds in 10 days! Today, my fibromyalgia is almost gone. I feel so grateful, I had to thank you and the Bragg Company for the most awesome, precious, enlightening and compelling translation job I ever did ! God Bless Bragg Crusades! – Ivannia, Costa Rica

Change your thoughts and you change your world. – Norman Vincent Peale

Praises and Testimonials for The Bragg Healthy Lifestyle

I am following the Bragg Healthy Lifestyle which I heard of through a friend. Your books are motivators and have blessed my health and life and are making perfect gifts for my family and friends. – Delphine, Singapore

---

I love Bragg Books, especially "The Miracle of Fasting". They are so popular and loved in Russia and Ukraine. I give thanks for my health and my super energy. I won famous Honolulu Marathon with all-time women's record! – Lyubov Morgunova, Champion Runner, Moscow, Russia

---

Thanks to you and your wonderful father for your guidance and teaching over the years. What a great gift you and your father have provided for us all through your Bragg Health Books and wonderful Bragg Health Products. Your Fasting and Vinegar books have improved my life immensely. I've lost 30 lbs. and feel years younger. At 67 youthful years, I give thanks for the great benefits of health I enjoy because of the work you and your father have so generously dedicated your lives too!! Wishing you every blessing under the Sun. –Captain Wes Herman (retired) Santa Barbara County Fire Dept.

I thank Paul Bragg for his Health Pioneering and Crusading. Dr. Bragg paved the way for our 100% healthy principles and inspired me to start the Good Earth Restaurants. I am a Bragg Product user and enthusiast. – Bill Galt, CA

In 1975 I was diagnosed with coronary heart disease. I followed the Free Bragg Exercise Classes and Health Lectures at Fort DeRussy lawn, Waikiki Beach, 6 days a week. Years have passed and I am going strong and healthy, thanks to The Bragg Healthy Lifestyle. In 1930's my father had severe hip arthritis and hardly able to walk. He followed the Bragg Healthy Lifestyle, also daily made his Bragg Vinegar Drinks and he cured his arthritis.
– Helen Risk, RN, Hawaii

Praises and Testimonials for The Bragg Healthy Lifestyle

After four weeks on Bragg Vinegar, my cholesterol went from 260 to 193. My PSA went from 4.4 to 3.6, it has not been that low since 1998. I was not on any other diet. It's amazing! Thank you. – Tom Reardon, MA

I started taking Bragg ACV and within days I noticed that my blood pressure lowered to 108/74. It is unbelievable! Please continue to spread health to our needed world! – Dr. Qasim Hussain Shah, Malaysia

I had 99% blockage in my carotid artery and was scheduled for surgery. I read "Bragg Apple Cider Vinegar" and "Super Power Breathing" book and started drinking Bragg Vinegar Drink!!! My Doctor says my artery is now "zero" blocked and my blood pressure and cholesterol levels are perfect. Huge Miracles! Thank You! – Joseph Gajdosz, NY

I give thanks to Health Crusaders Paul Bragg and daughter Patricia for their dedicated years of service spreading health as our Lord wants us healthy! It's made a great difference in my life and millions worldwide. – Pat Robertson, Host CBN "700" Club

I was diagnosed with diabetes and had high sugar levels. After following Bragg for 6 months, now I am insulin free and healthier than I have been for the last 15 years. My wife, three children and I are now healthy vegetarians living the Bragg Healthy Lifestyle. Results have been amazing. We thank You. – Dennis Urbans, Australia

Smile at yourself, smile at your wife, smile at your husband, smile at your children, smile at each other – it doesn't matter who it is – and that will help you grow in greater love for each other. - Mother Teresa

Man's precious breath is the gift of life from God.
With the care and nurturing of this life gift, all health and wisdom is ours.

Praises and Testimonials for The Bragg Healthy Lifestyle

I have been using Bragg Apple Cider Vinegar since the "Hippie Days". I am now 72 and enjoy it everyday. I have gotten off almost all my prescription drugs and I got your Bragg books out from years ago. Thanks for what you and your dad did for the health of millions. Forty years ago doctors didn't believe that food had anything to do with your health. Look where we are today. Your dad must be looking down from heaven seeing the footprints he made on the life of millions. God Bless. – Sharon

After meeting you in Australia, I began using Bragg Apple Cider Vinegar every day and suddenly I gained extra energy and my blood sugar levels stabilized, I lost weight and my hair and skin now healthy and glowing. When my 9 year old daughter, a ballet dancer, got a corn and painful planter's wart, I treated both with Bragg's ACV. The problems disappeared and she healed with no scar! Incredible! When my 2-year-old caught an awful case of molluscum contagiosum, dermatologists wanted to burn or cut out the unsightly bumps. I tried Bragg ACV instead and within 7 days all of the papules went black in the centre and cleared completely. Within a month there was no sign, she had over 50 of these horrible bumps on her legs!! It was AMAZING!! Thank you! If I had just one item in my medicine cabinet it would definitely be Bragg's Apple Cider! Kindest Regards, – Jane Allen and Family, Chinderah NSW, Australia

The Bragg book "Miracle of Fasting" inspired me to become healthy, trim and fit. I've finished 8 Boston Marathons. I was an unhealthy 350 lbs. and now a healthy 150 lbs, lean, trim and now also a Health Crusader. – Dick Gregory

Exercise, along with healthy foods and some fasting helps maintain or restore a healthy physical balance and normal weight for a long, happy life.

Praises and Testimonials for
The Bragg Healthy Lifestyle

I had heard on Dr. Oz TV show that drinking a mixture of 1 Tbsp Bragg Apple Cider Vinegar, (with the "Mother,") mixed with 16 ounces of purified water would melt belly fat. After a few weeks my waist was slimmer. I am a runner and had stopped running because of pain in my knees. My knee pain went away while I was drinking my ACV drink. Also, the past 5 years my blood sugar level has been 111. Since I started my Bragg ACV drink routine my blood sugar level has dropped to 90. I went on vacation for two weeks to Europe and didn't take my Bragg's Apple Cider Vinegar drink. My knee pain returned. When I returned home I started drinking my Bragg's ACV drink to start cleansing my body again. My knee pain is now gone and waist is slimming down.
Thank You!!! – Gina Santoro, New Jersey

The Lord works sometimes in ways we don't expect. He chose to answer my prayer by leading me to your health books and way of living . . . thus my medical problems are GONE! I want to give thanks to God, and to you, Patricia and your father. It was the Bragg Health Books that converted me to Healthy Living . . . and I will never be the same again! Thank You and God Bless. – Jimmy Damianos, Florida

---

Apple Cider Vinegar is the icing on the cake – a must read book! I had always heard about ACV . . . everyone in the world should be drinking this on a daily basis! The book is extremely informative and delightful to read. It answers all your questions and then some. Patricia and Paul's books have changed my life!!! – Dr. Steven Gibb

---

Your products are great. I have been using Bragg Apple Cider Vinegar and Liquid Aminos for years. I would never consider using soy sauce ever again! I use Bragg's in cooking all the time. Thanks for great health products. Keep up Health Crusading. – Glenda Berkley, Massachusetts

---

A fool thinks he needs no advice, but a wise man listens to others. – Proverbs 12:15

223

Praises and Testimonials for The Bragg Healthy Lifestyle

I bought and read the *Miracle of Fasting* e-book twice (plan to read it many more times). I feel blessed to have found your website, e-books and Bragg Healthy Lifestyle. Thank you so much. – Rick Cratty, Massachusetts

My parents, 91 and 86 are keeping youthful and enjoying Bragg Apple Cider Vinegar Drinks, it helps us with so many things!!! I appreciate your health teachings more than you know!!! – Barbara Magiley, Texas

In the past our family has had chronic health problems. Within the last year and a half God has shown us His Will for Healing and Divine Health. Our journey has included a healthy diet, some fasting and a complete change in lifestyle. We tried ACV and I want you to know that it is one of the most valuable changes that we have included in our lifestyle! It is terrific! I cannot express how good we feel! I am so thankful for every good thing that God has put before us – this journey, and every miraculous result and ACV is part of that. Thank you for sharing this wealth of health in Bragg Books. God Bless You! – Rhonda Jackson, Oklahoma

Thank you Patricia for our first meeting in London in 1968. When I was feeling my years, you gave me your "Miracle of Fasting" Book – it got me exercising – doing brisk walking and eating more wisely. You were a blessing God-sent and just when I needed to get more healthily recharged for Crusading. – Reverend Billy Graham • *www.billygraham.org*

Do not go where the path may lead. Go instead where there is no path, and thus leave a trail. – Ralph Waldo Emerson

A truly good book teaches me better than to just read it, I must soon lay it down and commence living in its wisdom. What I began by reading, I must finish by acting! – Henry David Thoreau

There is no thrill quite like doing something you didn't know you could. – Marjorie Holmes (find her books on Amazon.com)

"You change your life by changing your heart." – Max Lucado

Super Power BREATHING
For Super Energy, High Health & Longevity

Index

A teacher for the day can be a guiding light for a lifetime!

Bragg Books are silent health teachers – never tiring, ready night or day to help you help yourself to health! Our books are written with love and a deep desire to guide you to living a healthy lifestyle. – Dr. Patricia Bragg, Pioneering Health Crusader

Anyone who stops learning is old – whether 20 or 80. Anyone who keeps learning stays more youthful. Greatest thing in life is to keep your mind and heart young! – Henry Ford

"I conceive that a knowledge of books is the basis on which all other knowledge rests." – George Washington, 1st U.S. President, 1789-1797

With every new day comes new strength and new thoughts. – Eleanor Roosevelt

*Man's precious breath is the gift of life from God.
With the care and nurturing of this life gift, all health and wisdom is ours.*

Love is the sun shining in us to sparkle our lives and others! – Dr. Patricia Bragg

Wherever there is a human being, there is an opportunity for kindness. – Seneca

There's a positive side and a negative side and at every moment you decide.
–Sister Corita

Dream big, think big, but enjoy the small miracles of everyday life!

*Through our actions and deeds, rather than promises, let us display
the essence of love – perfect harmony in motion!* – Philip Glyn, Welsh Poet

*Kind words are a creative force, a power that builds up all that is good, and
energy that showers blessings upon the world.* – Lawrence G. Lovasik

We shall never know all the good that a simple smile can do.

Always do what is right – despite any public opinions.

Index

D

Daily Food Guide, 125
Daily Health Journal, 151
Dairy Products, *see Milk Products*
Dancers, 4, 189-190
Decongestants, 33, 37-38, 87, 93
Detoxify, 10-11, 32-34, 47, 54-55,
  119, 130, 134, 141, 207, 211
Diaphragm, 16, 19, 43-46, 50-51,
  54, 58, 62, 65-69, 72, 74, 80, 82,
  89, 169, 172, 184, 200-201, 210
Diaphragmatic Breathing, 18, 43-46,
  55-56, 69, 78, 189-190
Diarrhea, 32, 40, 184
Diet, 12, 14, 21, 33, 39-40, 58,
  84-85, 87, 92-94, 124, 126-127,
  129, 131-132, 134-137, 141,
  147, 153, 161, 182, 190, 206, 211
Digestive System, 8, 12, 47, 54
Distilled Water, 14, 32, 38, 57,
  76, 87, 94, 123, 125-126, 134,
  141-143, 146-147, 153, 166,
  176, 182, 207
Doctor Exercise, 183-194
Doctor Fresh Air, 177-182
Doctor Good Posture, 169-176
Doctor Rest, 163-168
Doctor Sunshine, 195-198
Drowning, 199-203
Drugs, 4-5, 12, 30, 49, 87, 94,
  165-166, 205, 211
Dyspnea, 83

E

Elimination, 22, 43, 45, 57, 147,
  151, 182-185, 191, 194
Emotions, 3, 15-17, 47, 56, 92, 174, 180
Emphysema, 6, 23-24, 30, 47, 59,
  84, 91-93, 114, 153, 158
Energy, 1-5, 9-10, 12, 14, 16,
  27-28, 47-48, 52, 54-55, 57,
  62, 65, 71, 77-81, 120, 123,
  126, 131, 151-153, 163-164,
  166, 168, 172-174, 178, 181,
  187, 189-191, 194, 207, 209, 211
Exercise, d, h, j, iii, 2-3, 7, 10, 13,
  31, 46-47, 52-54, 65, 85, 92, 94,
  98, 100, 108, 114, 119-120, 123,
  129, 151, 155, 162, 165-166, 170,
  172-174, 180-194, 198
Eyes, 12, 29, 35, 40, 48, 73, 77, 86,
  106, 109, 111, 130, 190

F

Fasting, 31-32, 57-58, 93, 134, 141,
  144, 146-147, 165, 174, 180-181,
  190, 211
Fatigue, 16, 49, 58, 70, 84, 99-100,
  154, 170, 175
Feet, 6, 31, 55, 57, 98, 140, 152,
  163, 169, 174-176, 185, 187, 211
Feldenkrais Method, 210
Filters, *see Air Filters/fans*
Flaxseeds, 88, 90, 125, 128, 130,
  133, 149 (recipes)

During your weekly 24 hour fast try to avoid criticizing anyone or anything!
Fill yourself only with loving, positive thoughts, not only on your fasting and
cleansing days, but everyday! Before you speak put your words to this test!
Is it good? Is it kind? Is it necessary? If not, don't speak! – Patricia Bragg, ND, PhD.

Habits can be right or wrong, good or bad, healthy or unhealthy, rewarding or unrewarding, powerful for good, or powerful for bad. The right or wrong habits and lifestyle decisions, actions, words and deeds are all up to you. Wisely choose your habits and lifestyle, as they can make or break you!
– Patricia Bragg, ND, PhD., Pioneer Healthy Lifestyle Educator

The future belongs to those who believe in the beauty of their dreams.
– Eleanor Roosevelt, First Lady of U.S., 1933-1945, husband President Franklin D. Roosevelt

Create highest, grandest vision for your life, because you become what you believe.
– Oprah Winfrey, talk show host, actress, producer, and philanthropist

Roses are God's autograph of beauty, fragrance and love.
– Paul C. Bragg, ND, PhD., Life Extension Specialist
Take Video Tour of Bragg beautiful Rose Garden on web: Bragg.com

Index

An Old English Prayer

Give us Lord, a bit of sun,
A bit of work and a bit of fun.

Give us in all the struggle and sputter,
Our daily whole grain bread and food.

Give us health, our keep to make
And a bit to spare for others' sake.

Give us too, a bit of song,
And a tale and a book, to help us along.

Give us Lord, a chance to be
Our goodly best for ourselves and others,
Until men learn to live as brothers!

Be kind to each other – You can work miracles with kindness.
A little kindness can make a big difference! – Saint Mother Teresa, 1910-1997

No matter what your sense of direction, you'll never lose your way.
Your angel will always keep you on the right path. – Suzanne Siegel Zenkel

Too often we underestimate the power of a kind touch, a warm smile,
a kind word, a listening ear, an honest compliment, or the smallest act
of caring, all of which have the potential to turn a life around.
– Leo Buscaglia, PhD., Author, Bragg Friend and Health Follower loves Bragg

Index

Smiles increase your face value! A genuine smile is love you give to yourself and others.

---

*There is no such thing as too many friends, just as there is
never too much happiness!* – Jean de La Bruyere

---

*May your mind forever sparkle like a star, your heart remain pure as new
fallen snow and your spirit forever sense the wonderment of a child.*
– Mary Summer Rain, Author – books available on *amazon.com*

*If I were to name the three most precious resources of life,
I would say books, friends and nature; and the greatest of these, at least
the most constant and always at hand is Mother Nature and God.* – John Burroughs

*A book is a garden, an orchard, a storehouse, a party, a mentor,
a teacher, a guidepost, and a counsellor.* – Henry Ward Beecher

All our dreams can come true – if we have the courage to pursue them.
– Walt Disney, famous Disneyland creator, Disney movies

*I am beginning to learn that it is the sweet, simple things of life
which are the real ones after all.* – Laura Ingalls Wilder, Author

*When we begin to trust ourselves more, the body begins to renew itself
and becomes healthier and filled with more life energy.* – Shakti Gawain

*A gift is pure when it is given from the heart to the
right person at the right time and at the right place
and when we expect nothing in return.*

Peace is not a season, it is a way of life.

V

W

Y

HAVE AN APPLE HEALTHY LIFE!

The future belongs to those who believe in the beauty of their dreams.
– Eleanor Roosevelt, wife of U.S. President Franklin D. Roosevelt, 1933 – 1945

*Create the highest, grandest vision for your life, because
you become what you believe.* – Oprah Winfrey

Self-discipline is your golden key; without it, you cannot be happy.
– Maxwell Maltz, MD – Author "Psycho-Cybernetics", Bragg follower we greatly admired.

*Breathing deeply, fully and completely energizes the body, it calms the nerves,
fills you with peace and helps keep you youthful.* – Paul C. Bragg, ND, PhD.

"You change your life by changing your heart." – Max Lucado

THE MIRACLES OF APPLE CIDER VINEGAR FOR A STRONGER, LONGER, HEALTHIER LIFE

The old adage is true:
"An apple a day keeps the doctor away."

- Helps promote a youthful skin and vibrant healthy body
- Helps remove artery plaque, infections and body toxins
- Helps fight germs, viruses, bacteria and mold naturally
- Helps retard old age onset in humans, pets and farm animals
- Helps regulate calcium metabolism
- Helps keep blood the right consistency
- Helps regulate women's menstruation, relieves PMS, and UTI
- Helps normalize urine pH, relieving frequent urge to urinate
- Helps digestion, assimilation and helps balances the pH
- Helps protect against food poisoning and even brings relief if you do get it
- Helps relieve sore throats, laryngitis and throat tickles and gargling cleans out throat and gum toxins
- Helps detox the body so sinus, asthma and flu sufferers can breathe easier and more normally
- Helps banish acne, athlete's foot, soothes burns, sunburns
- Helps prevent itching scalp, baldness, and dry hair
- Helps banish dandruff, rashes, and shingles
- Helps fight arthritis and helps remove crystals and toxins from joints, tissues, organs and entire body
- Helps control and normalize body weight

– Paul C. Bragg, ND, PhD., Health Crusader, Originator of Health Stores

Our sincere blessings to you, dear friends, who make our lives so worthwhile and fulfilled by reading our teachings on natural living as our Creator laid down for us to follow. He wants us to follow the simple path of natural living. This is what we teach in our books and health crusades worldwide. Our prayers reach out to you and your loved ones for the best in health and happiness. We must follow these wise laws He has laid down for us, so we can reap this precious health physically, mentally, emotionally and spiritually!

HAVE AN APPLE HEALTHY LIFE!

With Love,

236

Braggs Organic Raw Unfiltered Apple Cider Vinegar with the "Mother Enzyme" is #1 food I recommend to stop heartburn, gerds, gas, indigestion and for maintaining body's vital acid-alkaline balance and digestion.
– Gabriel Cousens, M.D., Author, "Conscious Eating"

BRAGG "HOW-TO, SELF-HEALTH" BOOKS

Authored by America's First Family of Health
Live Longer – Healthier – Stronger Self-Improvement Library

Qty.	BRAGG Book Titles Health Science ISBN: 978-0-87790	Price	$ Total
	10 BRAGG Book Offer – Get Healthy, Live Longer Special – plus in U.S. Free S&H ... all 10 only 89.00		•
	(Please see next 2 pages for book descriptions)		
____	**Apple Cider Vinegar – Miracle Health System** – Over 9 Million in Print	9.95	•
____	**Bragg Healthy Lifestyle – Vital Living to 120** – Simple & Easy-to-Follow	9.95	•
____	**Build Strong Healthy Feet – Banish Aches & Pains** – Dr. Scholl said, "It's the Best"	9.95	•
____	**Back Fitness Program** – For a Pain-Free, Strong, Healthy Back	9.95	•
____	**The Miracle of Fasting** – Bragg Bible of Health, Physical Rejuvenation & Longevity	11.95	•
____	**Healthy Heart** – Keep Your Heart & Cardiovascular Healthy & Fit At Any Age	11.95	•
____	**Super Power Breathing – for Super Energy & Longevity** – Helps to Heal Asthma & Allergies	11.95	•
____	**Build Powerful Nerve Force – Increase Energy** – Eliminates Fatigue, Stress, Anger & Anxiety	11.95	•
____	**Water, The Shocking Truth – That Can Save Your Life** – Stop Fluoride! Learn Safest Water to Drink	11.95	•
____	**Bragg Vegetarian Health Recipes** – Over 700 Delicious, Nutritious, Healthy Recipes	13.95	•
	<u>**Bragg Books Below are Available in Spanish (Libros En Español)**</u>		
____	**Vinagre de Sidra de Manzana – Sistema de Salud Milagroso** – Más de 9 millones impresos	9.95	•
____	**Estilo de Vida Saludable Bragg – Vivir De Forma Vital hasta los 120** – simple, fácil de seguir	9.95	•
____	**Corazón Saludable Bragg** – Mantenga su sistema cardiovascular saludable y en forma a cualquier edad	11.95	•

TOTAL COPIES	Books also available as E-books – see bragg.com All 10 E-books available for $9.90.	**TOTAL BOOKS** $	•

Please Specify: ☐ Check ☐ Money Order ☐ Credit Card

Books Only: CA Residents add 8% tax	•
(S&H) Shipping & Handling	•

Charge To: ☐ Visa ☐ Master Card ☐ Discover

Month   Year
_____
Card Expires

VISA   **MasterCard**   **DISCOVER** NETWORK

CVV #: _____

_____
Credit Card Number

_____
Signature

(USA Funds Only)
TOTAL BOOKS $ •

USA Shipping — Please add $6 first two books plus $1 each additional book
~ **FREE S&H in U.S. 10 Book Special** ~
USA retail book orders over $50 add $10 only

International Shipping — For Int'l orders, please email us at: CustomerService@bragg.com or fax: 1-805-968-1001 with your order details for shipping quote.

_____
Name
_____
Address   Apt. No.
_____
City   State   Zip
( )
Phone   e-mail

BOF 116

All Book & Shipping Prices subject to change at any time.

"BRAGG HEALTH BOOKS ARE GIFTS FOR LIFE"

Gen. 6:3

3 John 2

– Jack LaLanne, "Bragg took me at 15 from Sickness to Super Health!"

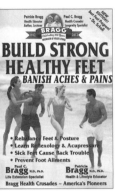

BUILD STRONG HEALTHY FEET
BANISH ACHES & PAINS

- Rebuild Feet & Posture
- Learn Reflexology & Acupressure
- Sick Feet Cause Back Trouble
- Prevent Foot Ailments

Bragg N.D., Ph.D.   Bragg N.D., Ph.D.
Bragg Health Crusades – America's Pioneers

978-0-87790-130-3 – $9.95

Learn how to banish aches & pains. Read about Reflexology, Acupressure and much more. Almost all of us are born with perfect feet. It's the abuse millions give their feet that makes them cry as they limp through life – "my aching feet are killing me!" Read this book!

The Bragg Foot Program is the best. I thank Bragg Books and their wisdom for my long, active, healthy life.

– Dr. Scholl,
Famous Foot Doctor

SUPER POWER BREATHING
FOR SUPER ENERGY
High Health & Longevity

- EMPOWER YOURSELF
- ENERGIZE YOURSELF
- RELAX YOURSELF

Paul C. Bragg   Patricia C. Bragg
N.D., Ph.D.   N.D., Ph.D.

978-0-87790-120-4 – $11.95

Breathing deeply, fully and completely energizes, calms, fills you with peace and keeps you youthful. Learn Bragg Breathing Exercises for more go-power and Super Health!

Thanks to Paul Bragg and Bragg Books, my years of asthma were cured in only one month with The Bragg Super Breathing and Bragg Healthy Lifestyle Living!

– Paul Wenner,
Gardenburger Creator

NERVE FORCE
Cure For Those Dull, Dragged Out, Hopeless, Helpless Feelings

If You Have:
Insomnia
Depression
Chronic Fatigue
Anxiety Attacks
Stress Overload

Suffer From:
Health Burnout
Mood Swings
Nervous Indegestion
You Need This Book!

Bragg N.D., Ph.D.   Bragg N.D., Ph.D.
Bragg Health Crusades – America's Pioneers

978-0-87790-093-1 – $11.95

Millions of healthy, happy followers have learned to control and increase their Vital Nerve Force Energy – The Bragg Healthy Way. Here's Prevention and Health Maintenance all in one book.

I have my life back after many years of chronic fatigue, fibromyalgia and clinical depression. I give thanks to The Bragg Health Books.

– Marilyn Mason

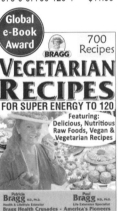

Global e-Book Award

700 Recipes

VEGETARIAN RECIPES
FOR SUPER ENERGY TO 120

Featuring:
Delicious, Nutritious Raw Foods, Vegan & Vegetarian Recipes

Bragg N.D., Ph.D.   Bragg N.D., Ph.D.
Bragg Health Crusades - America's Pioneers

978-0-87790-027-6 – $13.95

Enjoy the worlds finest health recipes for super health and high energy that you and your family will love. Over 700 Healthy Recipes for Health, Super Energy and Longevity. 336 pages filled with delicious raw and cooked foods, vegan and vegetarian recipes.

This book shows how to eat right with nutritious recipes to help maintain your body's health and fitness.

– Henry Hoegerman, M.D.

"I thank Paul Bragg and the Bragg Healthy Lifestyle for my healthy, long, active life. I love Bragg Books and Health Products."
– Jack LaLanne, Bragg follower to 96½ healthy, active years

"I have followed The Bragg Healthy Lifestyle for years and it teaches you to take control of your health and build a healthy future."
– Mark Victor Hansen, Co-Producer "Chicken Soup for the Soul" Series

"Thanks to Bragg Books for my conversion to the healthy way."
– James F. Balch, M.D., Co-Author of "Prescription for Nutritional Healing"

"Bragg Books have been a blessing to our family and the TBN family of loyal viewers."
– Evangelist Dwight Thompson, Co-Host TBN "Praise The Lord"

BRAGG BOOK SPECIAL ALL 10 ONLY $89. and in U.S. FREE Postage

If Bragg Books are unavailable in your area you may order:
on-line at: www.bragg.com or see Bragg booklist.
Bragg Book Special: All 10 books for only $89 Postpaid.

239

BRAGG ORGANIC APPLE CIDER VINEGAR

SIZE	PRICE		$ TOTAL	SIZE			$ Total	$ Amount
16 oz.	$4.09 each	Qty		16 oz.	$44.00 SPECIAL Case /12	Qty		•
32 oz.	$6.39 each	Qty		32 oz.	$69.00 SPECIAL Case /12	Qty		•
1 gal.	$20.79 each	Qty		1 gal.	$75.00 SPECIAL Case /4	Qty		•

FEDEX / UPS SHIPPING & HANDLING for USA	SPECIAL CASE – FEDEX / UPS SHIPPING & HANDLING for USA – Cost By Time Zone:	BRAGG VINEGAR $
16 oz. Add $10 for 1st bottle / $2 each additional bottle	16 oz: CA $15 • PST/MST $17 • CST $25 • EST $28	
32 oz. Add $12 for 1st bottle / $3 each additional bottle	32 oz: CA $20 • PST/MST $23 • CST $38 • EST $45	Shipping & Handling
Gallon: 1st Bottle: CA $12 • PST/MST $14 • CST $16	Gallon: CA $17 • PST/MST $22 • CST $34 • EST $40	
EST $18 + add $8 each additional bottle		TOTAL $ •

BRAGG LIQUID AMINOS

SIZE	PRICE		$ TOTAL	SIZE			$ Total	$ Amount
6 oz.	$3.79	Qty		6 oz.	$83.00 SPECIAL Case /24	Qty		•
10 oz.	$4.69 each	Qty		10 oz.	$51.00 SPECIAL Case /12	Qty		•
16 oz.	$4.99 each	Qty		16 oz.	$54.00 SPECIAL Case /12	Qty		•
32 oz.	$8.19 each	Qty		32 oz.	$90.00 SPECIAL Case /12	Qty		•
1 gal.	$29.99 each	Qty		1 gal.	$104.00 SPECIAL Case /4	Qty		•

FEDEX / UPS SHIPPING & HANDLING for USA:	SPECIAL CASE – SHIPPING By Time Zone:	BRAGG AMINOS $
6/10/16 oz: Add $10 for 1st bottle / $2 each additional bottle	6 oz: CA $12 • PST/MST $14 • CST $20 • EST $21	
32 oz: Add $12 for 1st bottle / $3 each additional bottle	10/16: CA $15 • PST/MST $17 • CST $25 • EST $28	
Gallon: 1st Bottle: CA $12 • PST/MST $14 • CST $16	32 oz: CA $17 • PST/MST $20 • CST $35 • EST $38	Shipping & Handling
EST $18 + add $8 each additional bottle	Gallon: CA $19 • PST/MST $24 • CST $38 • EST $45	
		TOTAL $ •

BRAGG ORGANIC OLIVE OIL

SIZE	PRICE		$ TOTAL	SIZE			$ Total	$ Amount
16 oz.	$13.39 each	Qty		16 oz.	$145.00 SPECIAL Case /12	Qty		•
32 oz.	$21.59 each	Qty		32 oz.	$233.00 SPECIAL Case /12	Qty		•
1 gal.	$69.99 each	Qty		1 gal.	$252.00 SPECIAL Case /4	Qty		•

FEDEX / UPS SHIPPING & HANDLING for USA:	SPECIAL CASE – FEDEX / UPS SHIPPING & HANDLING for USA – Cost By Time Zone:	BRAGG OLIVE OIL $
16 oz. Add $10 for 1st bottle / $2 each additional bottle	16 oz: CA $15 • PST/MST $17 • CST $25 • EST $28	
32 oz. Add $12 for 1st bottle / $3 each additional bottle	32 oz: CA $20 • PST/MST $23 • CST $38 • EST $45	Shipping & Handling
Gallon: 1st Bottle: CA $12 • PST/MST $14 • CST $16	Gallon: CA $17 • PST/MST $20 • CST $34 • EST $37	
EST $18 + add $8 each additional bottle		

BRAGG Apple Cider Vinegar, Liquid Aminos and Olive Oil are Foods and not taxable — TOTAL $ •

Please Specify: ☐ Check ☐ Money Order ☐ Credit Card

Charge To: ☐ Visa ☐ Master Card ☐ Discover

Month | Year

VISA   MasterCard   DISCOVER NETWORK

Card Expires

CVV #:

Credit Card Number

Signature

CREDIT CARD ORDERS

CALL (800) 446-1990 📞
8 am-4 pm PST • Mon.-Fri.
OR FAX (805) 968-1001

Business office calls (805) 968-1020.
We accept MasterCard, Discover or VISA phone orders. Please prepare order using this order form. It will speed your call & serve as your order record. Hours: 8 am to 4 pm Pacific Time, Mon. thru Fri.
• Web: www.bragg.com • e-mail: bragg@bragg.com

Mail to: HEALTH SCIENCE, Box 7, Santa Barbara, CA 93102 USA
Please Print or Type – Be sure to give street & house number to facilitate delivery.

Name

Address _____ Apt. No.

City _____ State _____ Zip

Phone ( ) _____ e-mail _____   BOF 116

| Bragg Health Products available most Health Stores & Grocery Health Depts Nationwide | 241 |

*All Product & Shipping Prices subject to change at any time.

6 BRAGG HEALTHY SALAD DRESSINGS & MARINADES

Bragg Organic POMEGRANATE VINAIGRETTE: Great-tasting, tangy, low-calorie, fat-free dressing for salads and flavorful seasoning for vegetables.

Bragg Organic APPLE CIDER VINAIGRETTE: It's great-tasting, zesty fat-free dressing for salads and flavorful seasoning for your favorite vegetables. Made with world famous Bragg Organic Apple Cider Vinegar.

2 NEW DELICIOUS DRESSINGS & MARINADES

HAWAIIAN Organic Dressing & Marinade: Brings Taste of Aloha to salads, veggies & stir-frys. Unlock Hawaiian secret flavors you will love.

BRAGGBERRY Organic Dressing & Marinade: New taste treats with Blueberries, Raspberries, Acai, Goji & Grape – powerful antioxidants!

GINGER & SESAME: Based on delicious flavors of famous Bragg Aminos & Ginger's sweet, tangy taste. Also great on veggies!

BRAGG VINAIGRETTE: Makes salad special with tasty, tangy flavor. Zesty blend of Bragg Apple Cider Vinegar and Bragg Organic Olive Oil, Bragg Liquid Aminos, garlic, onion, honey and delicious organic herbs.

America's Healthiest All-Purpose Seasonings

BRAGG SPRINKLE
ORGANIC 24 HERBS & SPICES

This old favorite is now available again. Bragg Sprinkle was created in 1931 by Paul C. Bragg, Health Pioneer & Originator Health Food Stores. Organic Sprinkle adds new healthy, delicious flavors to most recipes & meals. It's salt-free with no additives, preservatives or fillers.

BRAGG ORGANIC KELP SEASONING

This original Organic Kelp Seasoning is made from sun-dried Sea Kelp from pristine Atlantic Ocean waters combined with 24 all organic herbs and spices. It's a healthy, delicious seasoning for almost all recipes and meals and is specially suited for low-sodium diets.

BRAGG Delicious Nutritional Yeast Seasoning

Nutritionally designed to help meet nutritional needs of vegetarians, vegans and anyone wanting a good source of B12, B-Complex Vitamins. It's "cheese-like" flavor is a healthy delicious topping for most foods.

- Gluten-Free • Non-GMO
- No Salt • No Sugar • No Dairy
- No Artificial Colors & No Preservatives
- No Brewery Products
- No Candida Albicans
- All Vegetarian & Kosher Certified

242

BRAGG SPRINKLE – 24 Herbs & Spices Seasoning

SIZE PRICE	$ TOTAL	SIZE		$ Total	$ Amount
1.5 oz. $4.99 each **Qty**		1.5 oz. $54.00 SPECIAL Case /12 **Qty**			•
FEDEX / UPS SHIPPING & HANDLING for USA: Add $10 for 1st 3 bottles / $2 each additional bottle		SPECIAL CASE – FEDEX / UPS SHIPPING & HANDLING for USA – Cost By Time Zone: CA $10 • PST/MST $10 • CST $12 • EST $15	BRAGG SPRINKLE $		•
			Shipping & Handling		•
			TOTAL $		•

BRAGG ORGANIC SEA KELP

SIZE PRICE	$ TOTAL	SIZE		$ Total	$ Amount
2.7 oz. $4.99 each **Qty**		2.7 oz. $54.00 SPECIAL Case /12 **Qty**			•
FEDEX / UPS SHIPPING & HANDLING for USA: Add $10 for 1st 3 bottles / $2 each additional bottle		SPECIAL CASE – FEDEX / UPS SHIPPING & HANDLING for USA – Cost By Time Zone: CA $10 • PST/MST $10 • CST $12 • EST $15	BRAGG SEA KELP $		•
			Shipping & Handling		
			TOTAL $		•

BRAGG NUTRITIONAL YEAST

SIZE PRICE	$ TOTAL	SIZE		$ Total	$ Amount
4.5 oz. $6.69 each **Qty**		4.5 oz. $73.00 SPECIAL Case /12 **Qty**			•
FEDEX / UPS SHIPPING & HANDLING for USA: Add $10 for 1st 3 bottles / $2 each additional bottle		SPECIAL CASE – FEDEX / UPS SHIPPING & HANDLING for USA – Cost By Time Zone: CA $10 • PST/MST $10 • CST $12 • EST $15	BRAGG YEAST $		•
			Shipping & Handling		•
			TOTAL $		•

BRAGG SALAD DRESSINGS

ALL DRESSINGS & MARINADES: 12 oz. – $6.49 each or $35 SPECIAL case / 6 $ Total $ Amount

Ginger & Sesame	**Qty**		Bragg Hawaiian	**Qty**		
Bragg Vinaigrette	**Qty**		Apple Cider Vinaigrette	**Qty**		•
BraggBerry	**Qty**		Pomegranate Vinaigrette	**Qty**		
FEDEX / UPS SHIPPING & HANDLING for USA: Add $10 for 1st bottle / $2 each additional bottle		SPECIAL CASE – FEDEX / UPS SHIPPING & HANDLING for USA – Cost By Time Zone: CA $11 • PST/MST $12 • CST $14 • EST $16	BRAGG DRESSINGS $		•
			Shipping & Handling		•
BRAGG Sprinkle, Sea Kelp, Yeast and Dressings are Foods and not taxable			TOTAL $		

Please Specify: ☐ Check ☐ Money Order ☐ Credit Card

Charge To: ☐ Visa ☐ Master Card ☐ Discover

Month   Year

VISA   **MasterCard**   **DISCOVER**

Card Expires

_____

Credit Card Number

CVV #: _____

Signature

CREDIT CARD ORDERS
CALL (800) 446-1990 ☎
8 am-4 pm PST • Mon.-Fri.
OR FAX **(805) 968-1001**

Business office calls (805) 968-1020.
We accept MasterCard, Discover or VISA phone orders. Please prepare order using this order form. It will speed your call & serve as your order record. Hours: 8 am to 4 pm Pacific Time, Mon. thru Fri.
• Web: www.bragg.com • e-mail: bragg@bragg.com

Mail to: **HEALTH SCIENCE, Box 7, Santa Barbara, CA 93102 USA**
Please Print or Type – Be sure to give street & house number to facilitate delivery.

Name _____

Address _____ Apt. No. _____

City _____ State _____ Zip _____ BOF 116

Phone (___) _____ e-mail _____

Bragg Health Products available most Health Stores & Grocery Health Depts Nationwide

243

All Product & Shipping Prices subject to change at any time.

~ Please call stores first and if unavailable in your area use order form to copy and use ~

BRAGG ORGANIC APPLE CIDER VINEGAR DRINKS

ALL APPLE CIDER VINEGAR DRINKS: 16 oz. – $2.59 each or $28 SPECIAL case / 12 $ Total $ Amount

Original ACV & Honey	Qty	Grape-Acai	Qty	•
Ginger Spice	Qty	Limeade	Qty	•
Apple-Cinnamon	Qty	Pomegranate & Goji	Qty	•

SHIPPING CHART FOR ACV DRINKS

number of bottles	CA	PST/MST	CST	EST
1-2 bottles	$9.00	$9.00	$10.00	$15.00
3-4 bottles	$9.00	$9.00	$12.00	$15.00
5-6 bottles	$10.00	$10.00	$14.00	$15.00
7-12 bottles	$12.00	$15.00	$23.00	$28.00
SPECIAL Case/12	$12.00	$15.00	$23.00	$28.00

BRAGG ACV DRINKS $ •
Shipping & Handling •
TOTAL $ •

Please call around to Health & Grocery Stores first, because many stores are now selling Bragg Products or check web: bragg.com

BRAGG ORGANIC APPLE CIDER VINEGAR and ORGANIC HONEY CONCENTRATE BLEND

SIZE	PRICE	$ TOTAL	SIZE		$ Total	$ Amount
16 oz.	$8.99 each	Qty	16 oz.	$97.00 SPECIAL Case /12	Qty	•
32 oz.	$15.99 each	Qty	32 oz.	$172.00 SPECIAL Case /12	Qty	•

FEDEX / UPS SHIPPING & HANDLING for USA:
16 oz: Add $10 for 1st bottle / $2 each additional bottle
32 oz: Add $12 for 1st bottle / $3 each additional bottle

SPECIAL CASE (12) – FEDEX / UPS
SHIPPING & HANDLING – By Time Zone:
16 oz: CA $15 • PST/MST $17 • CST $25 • EST $30
32 oz: CA $22 • PST/MST $28 • CST $42 • EST $50

BRAGG BLEND $ •
Shipping & Handling
TOTAL $ •

BRAGGZYME – Systemic Enzyme

SIZE	PRICE	$ TOTAL	SIZE		$ Total	$ Amount
120 cap	$43.95	Qty	120 cap	$483.00 SPECIAL Case /12	Qty	•

No Shipping Charges on Braggzyme

BRAGG APPLE CIDER VINEGAR DRINKS & BRAGG HONEY CONCENTRATE BLEND are a food and not taxable!

BRAGGZYME $ •
Sales Tax for BRAGGZYME CA Residents ONLY add 8% TAX •
TOTAL $ •

Please Specify: ☐ Check   ☐ Money Order   ☐ Credit Card

Charge To: ☐ Visa   ☐ Master Card   ☐ Discover

VISA   MasterCard   DISCOVER

Month Year
Card Expires

CVV #:

Credit Card Number

Signature

Mail to: **HEALTH SCIENCE, Box 7, Santa Barbara, CA 93102 USA**
Please Print or Type – Be sure to give street & house number to facilitate delivery.

Name

Address   Apt. No.

City   State   Zip   BOF 116

Phone (   )   e-mail

Bragg Health Products available most Health Stores & Grocery Health Depts Nationwide   245

*All Product & Shipping Prices subject to change at any time.

Send for Free Health Bulletins

Patricia wants to keep in touch with you, your relatives and friends about the latest Health, Nutrition and Longevity Discoveries. Please enclose one stamp for each USA name listed or visit *www.bragg.com* and sign up on-line for literature.

With Blessings of Health, Peace, Love and Thanks

Patricia

Please make copy, then print clearly and mail to:

BRAGG HEALTH CRUSADES, Box 7, Santa Barbara, CA 93102

Name

Address   Apt. No.

                                    State   Zip

Phone (   )   e-mail

Name

Address   Apt. No.

City   State   Zip

Phone (   )   e-mail

Name

Address   Apt. No.

City   State   Zip

Phone (   )   e-mail

Name

Address   Apt. No.

City   State   Zip

Phone (   )   e-mail

Name

Address   Apt. No.

City   State   Zip

Phone (   )   e-mail

Bragg Health Crusades spreading health worldwide since 1912

Paul C. Bragg, Father of the Health Movement in America, had vision and dedication. This dynamic Health Crusader for worldwide health and fitness is responsible for more *firsts* in the history of the Health Movement than any other individual.

Bragg's amazing pioneering achievements the world now enjoys:

- Bragg originated, named and opened the first Health Food Store in America.
- Bragg Health Crusades pioneered the first Health Lectures across America and he inspired followers to open Health Food Stores across America and then worldwide.
- Bragg was first to introduce pineapple juice, then tomato juice and smoothies to America.
- He introduced Juice Therapy in America by importing the first hand-juicers.
- He was the first to introduce and distribute honey and date-sugar nationwide.
- He pioneered Radio Health Programs from Hollywood 3 times daily in 1920's - 1940's.
- Bragg and daughter Patricia pioneered a Health TV show from Hollywood to spread The Bragg Health Crusade on their show, *Health and Happiness*. It included exercises, health recipes, visual demonstrations and guest appearances by famous, health-minded people.
- Bragg opened the first health restaurants and the first health spas in America.
- He created and produced the first health products and then made them available nationwide: herbal teas, health beverages and oils, seven-grain cereals and crackers, vitamins, calcium and mineral supplements, wheat germ, whey, digestive enzymes from papaya, sundried fruits, raw nuts, herbs and kelp seasonings, amino acids from soybeans, healthy candy bars, health cosmetics, etc. Bragg inspired others to follow (Schiff, Gardenburger, Shaklee, TwinLabs, Trader Joe's, GNC, Herbalife, etc.) and now there are thousands of health stores & health items available worldwide!

Crippled by TB as a teenager, Bragg developed his own eating, breathing and exercising program to rebuild his body into an ageless, tireless, pain-free citadel of glowing, super health. He excelled and won events in running, swimming, biking, weight lifting and tennis. He made an early pledge to God, in return for his renewed health, to spend the rest of his life showing others the road to super health. He honored his pledge! Paul Bragg's health pioneering made a difference worldwide!

A legend and beloved Health Crusader to millions, Bragg was the inspiration and personal health and fitness advisor to top Olympic Stars from 4 time swimming Gold Medalist Murray Rose, to 4 time track Gold Medalist Betty Cuthbert of Australia, his relative pole-vaulting Gold Medalist Don Bragg, and countless others. The Hulk, Lou Ferrigno, went from puny to super shape. Jack LaLanne, the original TV Fitness King, says, *"Bragg saved my life at age 15 when I attended the Bragg Crusade in Oakland, California."* From the earliest days, Bragg advised the greatest Hollywood Stars and Giants of American Business, JC Penney, Del E. Webb, Dr. Scholl and Conrad Hilton are just a few who he inspired to long, successful, healthy, active lives!

Dr. Paul C. Bragg changed the lives of millions worldwide in all walks of life with the Bragg Health Crusades, Health Books and Products, Radio and TV appearances. (See and hear Dr. Paul C. Bragg on web: *www.bragg.com*)

PATRICIA BRAGG, N.D., Ph.D.
Health Crusader & Angel of Health & Healing

Author, Lecturer, Nutritionist, Health & Lifestyle Educator to World Leaders, Hollywood Stars, Singers, Athletes, etc. & Millions

Patricia is a 100% Health Crusader with a lifetime dedication passion like her father, Paul C. Bragg, world renowned health authority. Patricia has won international fame and awards. She conducts Bragg Health & Fitness Seminars & Lectures for Conventions & Schools, Women's, Men's, Youth & Church Groups worldwide. She promotes Bragg Healthy Lifestyle Living & "How-To, Self-Health" Books on Radio & TV Talk Shows throughout the English-speaking world. Consultants to Presidents & Royalty, to Stars of Stage, Screen & TV & to Champion Athletes, Patricia & her father co-authored The Bragg Health Library of Instructive, Inspiring Books that promote a Healthier Lifestyle, for a long, healthy, happy life.

Patricia herself is the symbol of health, perpetual youthfulness & natural femininity, radiant & super energy! She is a living & sparkling example of her & her father's Bragg Healthy Lifestyle & this she loves sharing worldwide.

A fifth-generation Californian on her mother's side, Patricia was reared by The Bragg Natural Health Method from infancy. In school, she not only excelled in athletics, she won honors for her studies & counseling. She is an accomplished musician & dancer, tennis player & mountain climber. Patricia is a popular gifted Health Teacher, a dynamic personality & perfect Talk Show Guest on Radio & TV Shows where she regularly spreads the simple, easy-to-follow Bragg Healthy Lifestyle for everyone of all ages. Patricia's been on the covers of many magazines as her health message is needed & well received by millions.

Man's body is his vehicle through life, his earthly temple & the Creator wants us filled with joy & health for a long, fulfilled life. The Bragg Crusades of Health & Fitness (3 John 2) has carried her around the world over 30 times – spreading physical, emotional, mental & spiritual health & joy. Health is our birthright & Patricia teaches how to prevent the destruction of our health from man-made wrong lifestyle habits of living.

Patricia's been a Health Consultant to American Presidents, British Royalty, to Champion Triathletes *(Patricia wrote 600 page Tri-Health Fitness Manual)*, Betty Cuthbert, Australia's "Golden Girl" (16 world records & 4 Olympic track star gold medals), & New Zealand's Allison Roe, Olympic Track & Triathlete Star. Millions follow Bragg Healthy Lifestyle like Hollywood's top Stars from Clint Eastwood to ever-youthful singing group – The Beach Boys, to Metropolitan Opera Singing Stars & top Ballet Stars, etc. Patricia's message is of worldwide appeal & well received by people of all ages, nationalities & walks-of-life. Those who follow The Bragg Healthy Lifestyle & attend Bragg Crusades worldwide are living testimonials like super athlete, Jack LaLanne, who at age 15 went from sickness to Total Fitness & Health to 96!

Patricia inspires you to Renew, Rejuvenate and Revitalize your Life with "The Bragg Healthy Lifestyle" Books and Health Crusades worldwide. Millions have benefitted from these life-changing events with a longer, healthier, happier life! She loves to share with your community, organization, church groups and conventions, etc. She is a perfect radio and TV talk show guest to spread the message of healthy lifestyle living. See and hear Patricia on web: *bragg.com* or on *YouTube.com/PatriciaBragg*. For radio and TV interviews, lecture requests call 1-800- 446-1990 or e-mail: **patricia@bragg.com**

248 BRAGG HEALTH CRUSADES, Box 7, Santa Barbara, CA 93102, USA